DENTAL ROENTGENOLOGY

BY

LeROY M. ENNIS, D.D.S.

ASSISTANT PROFESSOR OF ROENTGENOLOGY IN THE THOMAS W. EVANS MUSEUM AND DENTAL
INSTITUTE SCHOOL OF DENTISTRY, UNIVERSITY OF PENNSYLVANIA; INSTRUCTOR IN
DENTAL ROENTGENOLOGY, IN THE GRADUATE SCHOOL OF MEDICINE, UNIVERSITY
OF PENNSYLVANIA; LIEUTENANT COMMANDER, UNITED STATES
NAVY RESERVE

THIRD EDITION, THOROUGHLY REVISED

ILLUSTRATED WITH 789 ENGRAVINGS

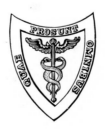

LEA & FEBIGER
PHILADELPHIA

TO ONE WHOSE SUPERIOR TECHNICAL ATTAINMENTS ARE ALWAYS GARBED IN MAGNIFICENT MODESTY, WHOSE HIGH HONORS BECOME HIM AS EASILY AS DOES HIS MANLY HUMILITY, AND WHOSE PRACTICE AND PERFORMANCE SQUARE ALWAYS WITH HIS ETHICAL AND PROFESSIONAL PRECEPTS—

ROBERT H. IVY, M.D., D.D.S., F.A.C.S.

PROFESSOR OF MAXILLO-FACIAL SURGERY, GRADUATE SCHOOL OF MEDICINE, AND OF CLINICAL MAXILLO-FACIAL SURGERY, THE THOMAS W. EVANS MUSEUM AND DENTAL INSTITUTE SCHOOL OF DENTISTRY, UNIVERSITY OF PENNSYLVANIA; COLONEL, MEDICAL RESERVE CORPS UNITED STATES ARMY

THIS TREATISE IS RESPECTFULLY DEDICATED

PREFACE TO THE THIRD EDITION.

THE first edition of this work was published in 1931, the second edition in 1936. During those nine years we have seen a growing interest in dental health, a greater mass interest among dentists in advancing dental health. Dental societies are holding more meetings, meetings more numerously attended, where they enjoy able discussions and well prepared papers covering every phase of dental research under the leadership of the most prominent savants in the medical and dental professions. This has brought greater progress to the profession with greater skill to the individual practitioner and has led to more intensive reading. Publishers of scientific treatises must be alert to include the latest developments and newest theories.

While acknowledging the urgings to hasten the completion of the manuscript of this third edition of Dental Roentgenology, it may be said with humility, albeit with no little feeling of appreciation, that the real incentive to carry on comes from the complimentary greetings and kind words with which the earlier editions received in every part of the world.

While adhering to the general form of presentation pursued in those earlier editions, I have made many justifiable revisions and many additions to the text. Improved equipment has been enumerated and described. In a separate chapter there has been considered the application of roentgenology to the youngest children, a discussion of deviations from the regular technique when required by peculiar conditions. Some better and clearer illustrations have been substituted where clearer illuminations of conditions under observation could be offered. Many additional illustrations aid in the interpretation of roentgenographic disclosures of both normal and pathological conditions. But the impressive result of the further study and research found in this edition is the confirmation and the demonstration that we continue to follow in even firmer reliance the very fundamentals of roentgenology and the techniques of application enunciated by the pioneers in that field.

This treatise is not to be considered the last word on the technique and interpretation of dental roentgenology. New theories and new applications are sure to follow, for roentgenology is a progressive science and, much as we have learned even in the past nine years, the proper interpretation of its results form a scientific study that is still in its swaddling clothes.

This book has been written to aid practitioners and students in acquiring and perfecting an effective technique in the exposure and development of roentgen films and to aid them in their accurate interpretation. It is based on the invaluable technical discoveries and theories of the pioneers in this field, on the clinical reports that followed them and on the author's personal experience resulting from continuous operating, teaching and interpreting in an atmosphere which demanded the best and accepted nothing less.

What is here recommended to others has been found effective in this active practice and has satisfied scientists and practitioners who have sought the most thorough information relative to dental and maxillary conditions. It has also provided an adequate basis for teaching dental students seriously bent on following dental roentgenology as a specialty in their profession. The purpose of this volume is to make this material available to everyone seeking a more thorough knowledge of the subject.

Since there can be no correct interpretation of roentgenograms of acute inflammation involving the teeth and their supporting tissues without an assured and accurate understanding of Pathology, the largest section of this book is devoted to Dental Pathology in its relation to Roentgenology. Interpretation must always depend on a thorough and systematic search for abnormal conditions and on their prompt recognition. Dental Pathology thus becomes an integral part of the study of Dental Roentgenology. It must be kept in mind, however, that this volume cannot comprehend any deep, definite treatise on pathology, and it makes no pretension of even an approach toward that goal. No dentist, it is assumed, would dare incursions into the danger-infested field of interpretation unless supported by years of study of oral pathology.

In order to make the book of equal value to dental students, to scientific dentists utilizing roentgenology as an aid to diagnosis and to Roentgen-ray technicians, it has been found necessary to curtail the discussion and explanations of the many topics introduced. The numerous articles cited and the recorded work of the pioneers will, it is hoped, open the doors to more intensive research to those who are so inclined.

The profound obligations of the author are hereby acknowledged for sympathetic coöperation and assistance of Robert H. Ivy, M.D., D.D.S., F.A.C.S.; Arthur Hopewell-Smith, L.R.C.P. (Lond.), M.R.C.S. (Eng.), L.D.S. (Eng.); Hermann Prinz, A.M., D.D.S., M.D., D.Sc.; E. Howell Smith, D.D.S.; Oscar V. Batson, A.M., M.D.; Jose Toledo, D.D.S.; and Clarence H. Goldsmith, LL.B., whose friendly criticism, untiring efforts, and sincere interest have been a constant source of help, in the preparation of this book. It is a further pleasure to thank Victor X-ray Corporation, Eastman Kodak Company, Ritter Dental Manufacturing Company and Lea & Febiger.

L. M. E.

PHILADELPHIA.

CONTENTS.

Introduction 13

CHAPTER I.

THE ROENTGEN-RAY TUBE 32

Construction of the Anode 36
Construction of the Cathode 38
Exhausting 38
Types of Dental Tubes 39
Electron Supply 40
Production of the Roentgen-ray 40
Electrons 41
    Outflow of Radiation, Time-distance Relation 42
    Amount of Radiation 42
    Quality 42
    Penetration 43
Elementary Terminology 43
Kinds of Electric Current Used 43
Roentgen-ray Current-voltage Requirements 44
    The Roentgen-ray Transformer 44
    Auto-transformer 45
    Stabilization 45
    The Coolidge Filament Transformer 47
    Rotary Converters 47
    Timers 48

CHAPTER II.

ROENTGEN-RAY DERMATOSIS 54

Course of Events in Chronic Roentgen-ray Dermatoses 58
Treatment 58
Idiosyncrasy 59
Radiation Test 59
Dental Fluoroscopy 60
Osteoradionecrosis 64

CHAPTER III.

INTRA-ORAL AND EXTRA-ORAL TECHNIQUE.

Roentgenologic Qualifications 67
Rules Governing Angulation 75
Intra-oral Roentgenology 77
Technique of the Occlusal Film 100
    Maxilla 100
    Mandible 105
Raper Bite-wing Film 108
Extra-oral Roentgenology 109

(9)

The Placement of Film in the Oral Cavity 124
    Maxillary Teeth 125
    Maxillary Molars 125
    Maxillary Left Premolars 125
    Maxillary Right Canine 126
    Maxillary Incisors 126
    Rules Guiding Placement of Film for Maxillary Teeth 126
    Mandibular Teeth 126
    Mandibular Molars 127
    Mandibular Premolars 127
    Mandibular Canines 128
    Guides for Placing of Film for Mandibular Teeth 129
    Film-holders 129
    Placement of the Occlusal Film 130
Gagging 130

CHAPTER IV

ROENTGENOGRAPHIC EXAMINATION OF CHILDREN

Basic Problems 132
Calcification of Teeth 132
Age at which Examinations are Made 138
Objective of Periodic Examination 143
Intra-oral Technique 148
Extra-oral Technique 153

CHAPTER V.

METHODS OF LOCALIZATION.

Stereoroentgenography 158
    Method of Exposure 162
    Root Fragments 167
Topographical Indications of Periapical Lesions 169

CHAPTER VI.

DENTAL ROENTGEN-RAY FILMS.

Dental Roentgen-ray Films for Intra-oral Work 171
    The Occlusal Film 172
    Inter-proximal Bite-wing Film 172
Dental Roentgen-ray Films for Extra-oral Work 172
    The Intensifying Screen 173
    Cassettes 174
    Static 175
    The Identifications of Roentgenograms 175
The Chemistry of Photographic Materials 176
The Chemistry of Development 177
The Chemistry of Fixation 180
The Chemistry of Reduction 182
The Chemistry of Washing 183
Temperature 184
Development 184
Practical Hints for the Dark-room 193

CHAPTER VII.

Routine Examination of the Oral Cavity.

The Electric Vitality Test 196
The Burton Vitalometer 198
The Thermal Test 201
Transillumination 201
Interpretation 202
Illumination 205

CHAPTER VIII.

Normal Anatomical Landmarks of the Teeth and Jaws as Seen in the Roentgenogram.

Landmarks of the Maxilla 209
The Nasopalatine Canals 210
The Maxillary Sinus 221
The Nasolacrimal Canal 252
Landmarks of the Mandible 253
Nutrient Canals of the Mandible 255
Tooth Development 267

CHAPTER IX.

Dental Pathology in Relation to Roentgenology.

Periapical Dental Lesions 274
   Proliferative Alveolo-dental Periostitis 277
   Chronic Rarefying Osteitis 277
   Chronic Rarefying Osteitis with Granulation Tissue 279
   Chronic Rarefying Osteitis with Suppuration 288
   Chronic Rarefying Osteitis with Cyst Formation 291
Lesions Involving the Investing Tissues of the Teeth 296
   Periosteal Abscess 299
   Condensing Osteitis 302
Pathological Conditions of the Dentine as Seen in the Roentgenogram . 306
   Adventitious Dentine 306
   Senile Dentine 307
   Calcareous Degeneration of the Pulp 308
   Dilaceration 308
   Gemination 310
Absorption of the Teeth 312
   External Absorption 313
   Internal Absorption 321
Hyperplasia of the Cementum 321
Sialoliths and Tonsilliths 321
Odontomas 327
   Epithelial Odontomas 327
   Composite Odontomas 342
   Compound Follicular Odontomas 342
   Extra-capsular Odontocele 342
   Cementoma 342
Torus Palatinus 342
Torus Mandibularis 344
Caries 346

Impactions 354
Residual Roots 364
Root-canal Fillings 368
Eastman Occlusal Film 377
Leontiasis Ossea. Osteomyelitis 384

CHAPTER X.

LOCALIZATION OF ROOT CANALS AND FISTULOUS TRACTS BY
               USE OF LIPIODOL 386
Technique of Introduction 391
    Root-canal Technique 391
    Cystic Technique 392
    Care of Syringe and Needle 392

DENTAL ROENTGENOLOGY.

INTRODUCTION.

I.

ONE wonders about the terrific suffering and high mortality rate that prevailed prior to the discovery and the diagnosis of appendicitis. It is given as a fact that cholera morbus, cramps, peritonitis and many other ailments were ascribed as contributing to deaths that really should have been diagnosed, would be today, as simple appendicitis. And the cures that were prescribed caused as much suffering as the ailment. It was, as today it seems to us as we look back, brutal, but a condition that is explained and excused as a result of allowable ignorance at the time.

One need not be bold to assert that the dentist caused as much suffering, probably more, and from an ignorance even more excusable, prior to the discovery of the roentgen-ray. When we contemplate the varied conditions related to us by patients, the few superficial indications from which we must chance a diagnosis, the justifiable hesitancy of any but the experienced oral surgeons to risk radical or comprehensive explorations, and the fact that we were limited so completely by mere clinical determinations in the treatment of assumed or presumed pathological conditions, it is remarkable that our guilt, or our responsibility, for myriads of progressing and chronic diseases of the teeth and jaw were not twenty times as great, and it is a tribute to the profession, to the care and caution and consideration and training of the average practitioner, that in the wake of our ministrations were not found more suffering than actually resulted.

The scientific dentist must concede that it is absolutely impossible to practise properly, thoroughly, without the assistance of roentgenology as an aid to diagnosis. There can be no discussion on that point. It is final. No factor in the practice of dentistry plays a more important part. And when we contemplate the few short years within which the science has been developed to the very high point of precision already attained, it is an outstanding compliment

(13)

to the pioneers in the field and to those who have continued the research work with the beneficent good attending; for the development and enlarging of the science of dental diagnosis and prognosis were accompanied by romance and drama that hold spellbound the student delving deeply into the heroic history of it all.

Theories born of bare experiences and meagre knowledge led to discoveries demanding and exacting martyrdom, even death, before truth unfolded itself for us and future generations. No part of the progress toward wider information about our physical and nervous system has been more important than the modern concepts of dental hygiene and therapeutics; for, while unknown and untold the real value must ever remain, modern dentistry has become the indispensable handmaiden of modern medicine.

Chance theories, lucky discoveries did not come from dreams; they flowed from minds immersed with myriads of ideas accumulated from the suffering of fellow humans, ideas that were born of kindness and an ardent endeavor to relieve such suffering, giving rise to speculation, and, in turn, through trials of flesh and spirit, through despair and many defeats, came the rays of light in the darkness as the setting sun often pierces the heaviest fogs besetting the bewildered mariner.

Some day, perhaps soon, as it should be, an inspired writer will seek out and narrate the tales of heroism lived by those seekers after science who have helped liberate mankind from the tortures of the days that knew merely bleeding for most ailments of the flesh, extraction for every toothache. And when such a book is written, those greater souls, those larger figures, whose researches allow us to know, to see, and to do what our predecessors in the profession dared not even guess, will have high place.

We must give full credit to Plucker for his continuous study of the green fluorescence of a discharge tube; the experiments, carried on for twenty years by Hittorf, Goldstein, Crookes, until, 1879, it was definitely determined that this fluorescence was caused by "something" coming from the cathode. This "something" could neither be found nor isolated sufficiently to be understood; but it could be labelled, even though the first discovery was mainly that a sharp shadow was cast upon the walls of the tube if certain substances, or articles, or objects, were placed within the tubes. Successively it was observed that the unknown "something," by them labelled "cathode rays," could be bent by a magnet, and that the rays travelled in straight lines, starting at right angles to the surface of the cathode, and, finally, when a concaved cathode was used, that the rays concentrated near the center of curvature and displayed heating properties and characteristics to excite phosphorescence in many substances.

Hertz and Lenard passed the rays through gold and aluminum foil, a particularly constructed vacuum tube having been devised for the experiment, and they declared the cathode rays similar to light rays. But other learned physicists opposed their conclusion because the deflectibility of the cathode rays led to a belief that the rays consisted of particles of matter charged with negative electricity and projecting from the cathode with great speed. Perrin, by catching the rays in a Faraday cylinder, did demonstrate that they carried a charge of negative electricity, following the conclusion of Thomson that the velocity of the cathode rays was less than the velocity of light.

The learned scientists of the world were engaged in experimenting with this yet unknown principle, each concluding and propounding theories of immense benefit though they differed widely in so many instances. But to Prof. Wilhelm Konrad Roentgen, of Würzburg, Bavaria, humanity owes honor and gratitude for discovering the most striking and outstanding property of the cathode ray. In 1895, while experimenting and searching for the invisible light rays, he turned on a low-pressure discharge tube completely enclosed in heavy black paper. Immediately, and to his surprise because unlooked for and not even in his contemplation, a fluorescent screen standing on a table some distance away was glowing brightly; and by interposing objects between the tube and the screen, shadows were cast on the screen. Tracing back the rays to their source, which was the region of the impact of the rays on the glass walls of the tube, he revealed that the rays were produced whenever and wherever the cathode rays encountered matter. Immediately he announced the significant information of the rays penetrating substances opaque to light, the degree of penetration depending upon the density of the substance, and the discovery that these rays could not be refracted or reflected, and could not be bent by magnetic or electric fields as could the cathode rays.

Peculiarly, it was an answer to the worry of many physicists who had been searching for an explanation of why unopened packets of photographic plates had become fogged while being merely held for use in laboratories; for then it became known that nearness to an active Crookes' tube had been causing the trouble.

Within fourteen days of the announcement of these rays that would penetrate solid substances impervious to light, Dr. Otto Walkhoff, of Braunschweig, Germany, had completed the first dental roentgenogram ever made. (Fig. 1.) This he accomplished by placing in his own mouth an ordinary glass photographic plate, wrapped in black paper and covered with rubber-dam, and submitting it to an exposure of twenty-five minutes—a dangerous experiment that indicates the recklessness of ignorance on the part of the pioneers in the field; and while the result of his attempt was crude and of no diagnostic value, there followed twenty years of tests and experiments that have brought our modern equipment, our better understanding of dental science, our beneficent assistance in reducing disease and suffering, and, not the least important, a realization of the dangers to both practitioner and patient of the unskillful handling of these powerful unknown rays. They are still an unknown quantity, just as they were when roentgen labelled them "*x*-rays."

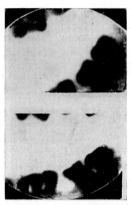

Erste Zahnaufnahme vom Lebenden

angefertigt 14 Tage nach der Veröffentlichung Röntgens im December 1895 auf einer zugeschnittenen photographischen Glasplatte von Dr. Walkhoff Zahnarzt in Braunschweig.

Fig. 1.—The first dental roentgenogram taken fourteen days after the roentgen-ray was discovered. This crude delineation of structural outlines demonstrated at once the possibility of producing clearer manifestations of structural composition and pathological processes under an advanced technique and with improved apparatus.

To those able, fearless, painstaking dentists, to Van Woert and Kells, who devoted their lives and forfeited much to develop for dentistry the discovery of Roentgen, to Raper, Simpson, Ivy, to Cieszynski who formulated many of the important basic principles of technique we now follow, and to others who blazed the trail that mankind might reap the benefit of their own travail and persevering devotion, the world is indebted beyond any calculation. They labored mightily and unselfishly, and the ramifications of their efforts insinuate themselves as memorials into every part of our present equipment, our study, our technique for the treatment of teeth. But the name and memory of the discoverer of these unknown or "*x*-rays" will be perpetuated as long as *x*-rays shall be used or mentioned; for they have borne and they will always bear his name and be known and designated as the roentgen-rays.

It was only shortly prior to the World War that roentgenology was entered into the curricula of our dental schools, and the great strides from the cumbersome equipment then used to the latest apparatus now available may be ascribed largely to the necessity of portable equipment required by the emergencies of that conflict. It is now possible for ever dentist to include a complete roentgen-ray apparatus in his office equipment.

Some have questioned the results of this availability, for there have been doubtful as well as positive results arising therefrom. The trouble is that many dentists consider themselves roentgen-ologists merely because they possess the apparatus. With equal justification every dentist who owns the necessary instruments might declare himself an oral surgeon, and we know the study and experience that are required before we consider anyone entitled to that eminent distinction.

Putting it straightforwardly, no dentist can qualify as a roent-genologist merely from sporadic experiments after a desultory course of reading and a superficial line of instruction at the hands of the equipment salesman, and yet there are many dentists who presume to do so. There lies a danger that needs no lengthy explanation. There must be a touch, a feeling, an incisive and decisive technique, an assurance that can come only with continued practice, an intensive experience, that the average occasional practitioner cannot possibly attain.

To make a thorough study of the theory of the roentgen-ray, the apparatus, the technique of using it, and the interpretation of the completed roentgenogram is no definitely small and circumscribed field. Rather it is a very large, and almost unlimited field if properly explored, and to attempt anything less than a full study of the field is doing things improperly. Impending danger lurks in the path of the unqualified or unprepared roentgenologist.

Notwithstanding the glib representations of salesmen that the absolute safety of their apparatus requires hardly any training upon the part of the operator, bear in mind that all types of apparatus are dangerous unless used with the most meticulous care. It

2

should be evident to the least scientific that, when rays are generated in a tube there must be some point of escapement for the rays to produce an effect upon the photographic emulsions, and if an effect upon this emulsion is produced there must necessarily be some effect upon any living tissues exposed to the rays, the greater the exposure either in time or number creating the greater effect; and the effect may be quite dangerous.

Another superficial observation is pertinent: the operator must realize that dental units are not constructed to have the penetrating qualities of the apparatus used by general roentgenologists; they are particularly designed for the special field of operation. And most general roentgenologists, it may be said advisedly, are not as well qualified in the special field governing conditions affecting the teeth as are those who devote their entire practice to that field. This conclusion has been forced upon those who have seen roentgenograms and read interpretations, great numbers of them, coming from both the general and the dental roentgenologist.

The roentgenologist treats with mere shadows, studies and interprets these light, unsubstantial shadows. Any misconception of their indications may be a blunder that wrecks happiness, health, and the opportunity for misconceptions arise from the lack of proper technique in the making of roentgenograms as well as from the lack of proper schooling in the interpretation of them. Ability to do both thoroughly is a mandate that science will not compromise.

II.

Not long ago there came together to consult a roentgenologist two men, Dr. Tweedledum, a dentist, and Dr. Tweedledee, a physician, each of whom held a seemingly good practice in his respective profession in a fairly populous community.

Presenting two very fair looking roentgenograms of the right mandibular region that showed in succession a full complement of teeth, and then a film indicating the recent removal of the second molar, they related the case: a young lady, aged twenty-one years, had been suffering from what the physician had diagnosed as some form of arthritis; the dentist made the roentgenograms; the film indicated to them a condition of the second molar that might have contributed to the condition; the tooth was extracted.

But the suffering of the young patient meeting no amelioration, it was determined to remove the first premolar which to both dentist and physician seemed to show a condition warranting the course.

The only obstacle to carrying out the plan was the protest of the tearful owner that the first removal effected no relief and, with no greater assurance from the projected second extraction, she was not going to undergo the immediate loss and the subsequent cross of a larger bridge for the balance of her life without better promise of when and where the extractions were to end.

Well, an easily arrived at interpretation of the film indicated no pathological condition to have justified the extraction of the first molar. To the very contrary, it showed a strong, normal structure with good, healthy pulp, free of caries and traces of degenerated tissue, abscesses, or doubtful physiological appearances, save a natural or, at least, no unusual calcification surrounding part of the apical region met hundreds of times in our regular practice.

One not pretending to superior attainments in the field could have interpreted the film. Yet that innocent and vital tooth would have been extracted save for the wise opposition of the patient.

But the more serious side of the situation lies in the fact that the second molar, which had been extracted in vain as far as the accomplishment sought by its removal concerns, was even a more perfect bit of tooth structure, its surrounding tissues pathologically unquestionable. The roentgenograms confirmed this deduction clearly.

This case typifies thousands encountered in any metropolitan city. Multiply the number by any figure in your imagination and you might approximate the woe that wallows in the wake of inaccurate interpretations of even ample roentgenograms and of faulty application following an interpretation of improperly produced films.

Thousands of cases there are where the less careful and the less trained observer attributes as a sign of infection shadows delineated on a roentgenogram that to the capable clinician show normalcy or, at most, the slightest deviation from the normal, but which indicate neither infection nor a condition contributing to infection. And perhaps a much greater number of cases there are where the practitioner fails to recognize shadows portending danger, fails to observe shadows of evident abnormalities that indicate infection or threaten at no distant time to result in or produce infection.

Following the trail of the wild orgy of extracting teeth indulged
so horribly a few years ago, there are still too many removals of
good and vital teeth by dentists who hold themselves out as capable,
and not only by the mercenary, commercial cult that sees in extraction the fatter return from the making and sale of appliances.
There is no argument with medical diagnoses thoroughly, scientific-
ally made; but physicians are still prone to blame teeth for all
human ills failing to respond to orthodox or inexpert medical treatment: and so the tooth that Dr. Tweedledum could not observe
was harmless, and that Dr. Tweedledee could not diagnose as
uninfected, comes out. And the plight of the poor patient is
pathetic, to apply no more condemnatory term when contemplating
the ignorance that permitted it.

But to the myriads of cases where flagrant ignorance of dentists
allows serious conditions of the teeth and tissues of the oral cavity
to persist for years without warning or attention, the only word
applicable is "tragic." In this year of grace no excuse is offerable
for thousands of infections remaining unnoticed until immediately
imperative surgical operations are required. The past ten years
have given successive suggestions as to the care of the teeth, ample
admonitions as to the dangers of neglect, have placed within grasp
the knowledge and the instruments through which to discover oral
conditions calling for treatment to protect health; and the dentist
who deliberately or carelessly refuses or neglects to employ every
known instrumentality and method to detect indicia of disease,
who sidesteps science because of an inability or an ineptitude to
keep abreast of the modern speed of progress, who continues following the hit-or-miss system of treating suspicious symptoms instead
of searching and treating the causes, who, in fine, is smugly satisfied with anything less than the fullest and most comprehensive
method of diagnosing the ills to which the constituent parts of the
mouth are subject—that dentist is unfair to the patient, unfair to
the public, unfair to the profession.

The oral surgeon views many cases that may not come within
the purview of general dental practice very often; but it would
surprise many were the surgeon to mention the number of cases
that might have been saved his scalpel and lancet had the dentist
but employed early the ordinary safeguards and methods of examination that lay as close to hand as do his elevators, or mirrors, or
explorers.

That a thorough, full mouth examination of every one seeking the services of the dentist is necessary has been proven by recent research and very specific confirmations of scientific theory; and to convince the patient of this is the inescapable responsibility of the practitioner. For where teeth exist or existed, there lies not only the safeguards of health but also, though so often deeply hidden, undiscerned dangers to health.

We understand now how in the unexplored and, except for curious, experimental surgery, well nigh unexplorable maxillary and mandibular structures lay for years undiscovered foci of systemic infection. We had wondered, pondered, guessed as to what undisclosed conditions might lie beneath the surface, often exploring just short of or just wide of finding anything of informative value. No clinical test revealed more than a justification for further guesses. And, when later, we noticed erupting from the tissues of an hitherto unsuspected area a condition dangerous and menacing, one which in growth and propagation consumed not only days, nor months, but years, we bemoaned our helplessness, hoped for knowledge to insure earlier recognition of danger signs, prayed science to provide us with better methods of diagnosis, better systems of determining the etiology of dental diseases. And through her handmaiden, through the heroic pioneers in all fields of dental science whose study, struggles, sufferings have made dentistry the honored and respected profession it has become, science answered that prayer. Science answered that prayer the fullest when Wilhelm Konrad Roentgen announced the discovery of the outstanding and striking property of the cathode ray, his own-named x-ray, with which, compared to the darkness wherein dentistry labored before this beneficent discovery, miracles of yesteryear are the common routine of our present practice.

Even the younger generation of the profession has seen the infancy and growth of this landmark, and thanks to the deep and scientific interest these younger men have evinced, the acceptance and the application of the roentgen-ray in general practice has proven the greatest boon that has come to a suffering civilization since the offering of anesthesia eased the severity of pain and prolonged the days of those who number among the honored names revered in history. Those now coming into the profession are recognizing the roentgen-ray as the very support that dental science has sought these many years, for it has proven the most accurate, the most dependable, the most truthful aid the clinician can summon when in doubt. The roentgen-ray is an aid, an aid of incalculable value, not a solely sufficient system of examination.

It is no pleasing commentary to review the difficulty encountered in securing the acceptance and the recognition of the value of the roentgen-ray by the older and more experienced members of the profession. Dentists, physicians, like some business men who feel their success measured by the income and are too satisfied to consider changing either methods or standards, cling to old ideas and old ideals, smugly unaware these are being relegated to the dust heap by the progressive and scientific world. Their preconceptions are rooted very deep, and a coddled inertia deters them from effort to understand the newer ideas that appear; but a few years hence will see them superseded in the estimation of the patients and the public by the younger men who are so keenly alive to the thrilling experiences that are making dentistry so important and so progressive a science.

For the past five years, each student entering Drexel Institute, Philadelphia, has been given a thorough and comprehensive medical and dental examination. Drexel Institute is a school comparing with the average smaller college, with students of the average age, average intellectual grasp, and of the average family connections and environments that attach to the general run of college matriculates of both sexes, for it is coeducational.

There has been a progressive change and improvement in the system of making these examinations from year to year, for, when originated, the plan comprehended merely the superficial clinical survey of the teeth, the idea being limited to a report on the more or less obvious conditions. The medical examiner had no small task in his own particular broad field: he was anxious to complete the examinations quickly; the number of students requiring attention influenced his desire to present his first report to the faculty at the earliest possible day so as to permit the formulation of plans to treat the subjects where dental or medical treatment was indicated as necessary. So it was ordered that only teeth creating justified suspicion be roentgen-rayed.

This was a system less than thorough, much less than adequate; and it required little argument to convince the medical examiner that his records would prove but a part of what his aim sought, for his final report confirmed the thought so fully that in the following year, and since then annually, a comprehensive clinical and roentgenologic full mouth examination has been made of all freshmen.

Bear in mind that the average age of these students is eighteen years, and that the questionnaire answered by them seems enlightening inasmuch as more than one-half replied that they had visited their family dentist for examination or for some specific treatment anywhere from within one month to six months just prior to their coming to college.

Eleven hundred and twenty-seven students formed the first group examined in 1931: males, 723, and females, 404. Only teeth suspected of periapical involvement were roentgen-rayed and of the 723 males examined only 200 proved free of caries under the rather superficial method then followed. Five hundred and twenty-three of these young men, ambitious, avid to attain an education, interested in preserving health, knowing the importance of a sound body to house a reasoning mentality, carried in their mouths the very well-springs of disorders and diseases, and of the presence of which they were totally unaware, that were as threatening as though the pure sources of the springs supplying the drinking water to their homes had been poisoned and polluted. Seventeen hundred and twelve cavities were discovered, not to mention 691 missing teeth that should have been replaced by substitutes to protect complementary vital teeth in danger of earlier degeneration were such action deferred unduly.

But only 294 of these 723 mouths were examined roentgenographically, because, to repeat, this method was applied only to those conditions indicating clearly a suspicion of periapical involvement: yet in these 294 cases there were disclosed 249 carious conditions that the mirror and other clinical instrumentation had failed to find.

Of course, a full roentgenographic examination of every mouth would have disclosed much that the employed method missed; but when approximately 85 per cent of the mouths examined under roentgen-rays exhibited conditions probably more dangerous than those treated by the family dentist just a few short months earlier, it cannot be a very happy thought for those same dental practitioners to contemplate, particularly with the possibility of these young students returning to the home towns with the report that Dr. Slipshod or Dr. Careless certainly overlooked some menacing conditions when pronouncing the patient perfect, with no oral condition to worry him or hinder his studies. And that is a threat that hangs over the heads of us all who are satisfied with only the merest clinical examination when surveying the teeth of a patient, and the threat grows larger each day.

The 249 definite carious conditions so discovered seems a sufficiently formidable justification of the roentgenographic examination; but in addition to these conditions, there were undetected by the clinical tests but discovered by the roentgen-rays in the same 294 mouths over 100 cases of granuloma, 1 cyst, 14 residual roots, 10 well developed cases of periostitis, and 38 plain instances of root absorption showing unmistakable conditions that should have been treated earlier.

Nor is it amiss to interpolate here a rather illuminating presentation of data showing the result of the roentgenographic examination of 25 young ladies studying oral hygiene. It is unnecessary to recite the educational qualifications these students are required to possess, but you may be assured they are ample. More, these students are certainly interested in the maintenance of their own teeth, the preservation of them, and surely since first contemplating the field they subsequently entered, they had probably looked after them more zealously than the average person looks after the teeth. Nor should we lose sight of the fact that many of the young ladies entering the course are the daughters, the sisters, or close relatives of dentists.

The mouths of these embryo oral hygienists should show an healthful state, a well attended set of teeth, an absence of infection and threatening growths. But the films, checked and rechecked with the greatest care and certitude, disclosed among the 25 students these conditions:

Caries	79	Condensing osteitis	1
Rarefying osteitis with granulation tissue	12	Perforated root	1
		Residual tooth	1
Impactions	13	Retained teeth	15
Root absorption	1	Missing teeth	41

With such impressive data collected from sources of knowledge of the value of hygienic and healthful oral conditions, we may pause to consider the gravity of conditions that might be found generally among the people in all walks of life were every inhabitant of our country subjected to a similar examination.

To revert to the result of the examination of the Drexel Institute students, but avoiding the detailed statistics pertaining to the 160 young ladies selected to undergo the roentgen-ray examinations, let it suffice to state that the roentgenographic survey showed a preponderant amount of infectious conditions, or pathological lesions that the clinical examinations did not disclose and never would have disclosed. So startling were the revelations among both the male and female groups that the school authorities determined quickly upon a complete full mouth roentgenographic examination for all future freshmen upon entering the college.

The examination of the class that entered in September, 1934, evidenced a greater prevalence of caries than the average found in earlier classes studied; but as to other conditions, practically similar proportions of infectious conditions were found as prevailed in preceding classes. The excess caries may be attributed to the economic conditions pressing heavily these past three or four years. Less than sufficient dental treatment might easily be an incident of the depression.

There is much to ponder over when reviewing the figures just offered. To approach the contemplation of conditions shown, it may easily be conceded that some of the students failed to adhere strictly to the truth when, during the examination, they were asked, "When did you last have the services of your dentist?" for quite too many replied, "Just prior to my departure for school," to deserve complete credence; for the plainly evident conditions observed through the mirror alone negatived many who so asserted and gave reason to suspect the credibility of some students.

But the veracity of the student becomes an issue only when considering with the finer point that leans toward the lesson the entire picture presents: if the conditions discovered among these students tower as glaringly and as threateningly to you as they seemed to the medical director and the faculty of Drexel Institute, how are we to protect the growing generation against similar danger? For it is logical to deduce that similar conditions exist all over the country. It is a fair assumption that even more pronounced would be the findings among younger persons not preparing for further studies, not undergraduate college students, not prospective oral hygienists. Among older persons, it may be ventured quite confidently, the infectious conditions that a complete examination would disclose might double or treble the number found among freshmen at our colleges and universities.

Every school and college will soon be doing what has been tried at Drexel Institute. Institutions not so well equipped within their own midst with forces to handle the examinations will require either a complete report from the dentist who last examined the student or a report from some reliable dentist in the college town. And a high degree of accuracy will be expected of these examinations, so dentists had better attend that discoveries so made tend not to the prejudice of the profession.

Data very illuminating may be drawn from the examination of one freshman class of 883 students at Drexel Institute when 27,398 teeth were under observation, and in 2797 of which caries were revealed. While the combined clinical and roentgenologic examinations disclosed 3634 carious areas, the clinical method found only 1662: the roentgen-ray found 1372; the roentgen-ray and clinical examinations agreed only in 237, which represents the comparatively small proportion, about 10 per cent of the carious conditions revealed, that was duplicated by the joint disclosures.

And if, however often you repeat a similar experiment on a large group of people your findings approximate such result, it is evident that to exclude either of these methods in examining teeth is to shirk a grave responsibility. Not only is there a responsibility upon the dentist to examine roentgenologically the clinically suspicious teeth, but that some attention should be given as surely to the entire mouth, the teeth and edentulous areas that exhibit no obvious suspicious appearances.

For no longer is the chief concern of the dental profession merely the repair, the replacement, the treatment of the obvious; the prevention of disease looms as largely important, and the sphere of the dentist embraces completely the minutely conceived function of prophylaxis. We know of systemic diseases originating in caries and other hidden oral putrefactions; we concede the deleterious influence of septic teeth and tissues; we dare not ignore an agency offering to disclose such foci of infection. To the contrary, we must have such an agency close at hand to locate and determine quickly where abnormal conditions exist. A roentgenographic outfit should be in every office. But not as an adornment; as a necessity.

No extravagant claims are advanced in favor of this conviction and none need be, for the self-evident truths proclaim to the world sufficient reasons, ample demonstrations of the incalculable value of the instrument. Of course the roentgen-ray misses many existing conditions. Caries may be so embedded in the pulp as to escape the penetrating eye of this miracle worker, and it will pass other danger spots that the explorer reveals; but without it you will miss granuloma, the chronic rarefying osteitis with granulation tissue, and you will miss many residual roots, and perforated roots, and a multitude of caries, not forgetting root fragments, diseased tissues, foreign substances in apical foramen, dentigerous cysts, salivary calculi, and other hidden dangers the discovery of which is the duty and function of each and every dentist pretending to the name and calling. Without the roentgenographic examination you will miss the assurance that comes from adopting the most scientific system of prophylaxis, of healing, of cure that modern methods demand we follow for the fullest protection of the patient.

The public schools, the radio, the newspapers have carried a widespread educational campaign covering dependence of health upon good teeth, and the preserving and retention of vital teeth. Hence the growing opposition to extractions unless as a last resort, the insistence of the patient upon roentgen-rays even after the attending dentist advises extractions, and many cases we know where the sufferer secretly seeks the roentgenologist before submitting to the exodontist to whom he had been referred, because we have a deeper understanding of the power of the roentgen-ray, of its attributes that penetrate beneath innocent appearing surfaces to delineate foci of infection that superficial surveys cannot depict. You notice how the advertising clique features the roentgen-rays in their publicity as a sign of advanced, modern method, and how their patients are harangued into believing every patient should undergo such an examination; and, in theory, you must concede, they have reason on the side of their argument.

With dentistry becoming the first support of modern medicine to stem the flood of systemic disorders viciously undermining mental and physical normalcy, it behooves the profession to put its house in order if it is to be the potent agency in preventing infection propagating into a virulence that may spell even untimely death; we cannt stand by supinely until bursting eruptions force the recognition of sepsis when the barest outlay of time and money would have detected the infection and could have aborted or removed it before it invaded deleteriously into deeper tissues and the blood stream.

Missionaries must preach the gospel of a full mouth examination for every patient, the records to be retained by the dentist, filed for future reference. The principles of prophylaxis commend the idea; it is the logical evolution of dental science toward decreasing destructive dental disease. But in the revelation of pathological lesions and the minute indication of their location, area and extent, there would also be a lessening of operative labor.

While monetary considerations hold no persuasive place in our discussion, it may be ventured that, the equipment once owned, the small cost of roentgen-ray films adds triflingly to the carrying charges of any office. Really, instead of an expense, the making and use of roentgenograms will show a profit and not a loss: for they contribute to building larger practices; they uncover conditions that would otherwise remain unrevealed and so untreated. Think of the time, trouble, worry, uncertainty saved when absolute certainty may be had for the mere asking, the mere concentrated attention called for in the study of roentgenographic technique.

No separate charge should be necessarily made patients for the service, whatever system of charges might be followed in offices, and this for several reasons: the service should be as incidental to the examination of a patient as is now the very first glance given a worrisome tooth or other trouble about which the dentist is consulted; it overcomes the natural reaction of the patient against individual fees for specific necessary treatments; it impresses patients that the service is the routine practice of the office, not extraordinary; and the resulting film is for your own knowledge and information and is not the property of the patient to display to his family and friends.

There seems no better reason to ask a separate fee for such an examination than, when making a clinical study, there would be charges for the use of pulp testers, transilluminators and for the wear and tear on engines and explorers. And right here it seems quite pertinent to quote from an article by Dr. L. M. Waugh, New York, appearing eighteen years ago in the *Dental Cosmos*, vol. 59, 1917, entitled "Radiology as an Adjunct in the Practice of Dentistry."

Dr. Waugh had sent to 325 outstanding dentists throughout the United States and Canada a series of questions which included the following:

"5. (*a*) Do you make a separate charge for each radiograph?
   Answered: Yes, 87; No, 62.

 "(*b*) If so, does the patient not sometimes question the need
   of several of a given case?
   Answered: Yes, 74; No, 34.

 "(*c*) If not in your own practice, do you believe this would
   be so in a great number of practices?
   Answered: Yes, 116; No, 28.

"(*d*) Would this not be overcome by having it understood that the necessary radiographs are a part of the service, and as such are not charged for separately but are included in the general fee.

Answered: Yes, 147; No, 8.

"(*e*) Do you find the time saved by radiodontic findings largely compensates for the time required in making them?

Answered: Yes, 162; No, 8."

The answers to these two final queries reflect an interesting attitude on the question under discussion; and when you appreciate that the questionnaire dates back to almost archaic days of dental roentgenography, and surely the infancy of the system, how could the returns be less impressive if a vote were taken at this time?

In over one-third of the dental offices in our country will be found some sort of roentgen-ray apparatus, whereas ten years ago the appearance of one was a rarity. The profession has learned that roentgenology need not be a specialty, and that, while demanding intensive application when studied as seriously as the subject warrants, and a profounder knowledge of many intricate phases of dental theory, physiology, pathology, etiology, as well as a technique akin to art, these very requirements are hardly more than every practitioner is supposed to possess in order to perform the usual functions the profession imposes. Capable dentists are counted upon to locate and diagnose pathological conditions of teeth, of the mouth, of the investing tissues, and it cannot be a soothing sensation to patient or dentist when for a mere roentgenographic examination a reference to some other dentist must be made. The astounding poignancy of this observation appears when noting how advertising quacks and impostors publicize this service, while the otherwise capable and ethical dentists admit unpreparedness in so abundant a field of endeavor.

You may assert that no criticism is levelled against the physician who refers a patient to a specialist, and the controversy created by the comment might be wordy before being fully threshed. But without the slightest disposition to avoid discussion, may it be ventured that the almost antipodean difference in the present-day scope and responsibilities of the neighboring though complementary but distinctly separated professions are the answers to the assertion. When analyzing the respective relations to the particular profession served, it is not easy to compare the pediatrician or the neurologist, or the psychiatrist, or the ophthalmologist to the roentgenologist. This passes by the thought of many physicians that too strongly has the impression become that the general practitioner has permitted himself to be erased from the medical picture; but knowledge of the terrific study and experience the medical man must possess to gain recognition as a specialist of highest repute, of the concentration he is required to give his special subject, of the never ending round of clinics he must attend, cannot be disregarded. But the degree of knowledge upon which the dental roentgenologist bases his prerogative to be conceded a specialist is hardly in excess of what every dentist is expected to possess. Surely the mere study incident to learning the application of that knowledge to the making of and interpreting of the roentgenogram lies within easy grasp. The capable dentist should not allow himself to be forced entirely into the background by the specialist, becoming a mere satellite of the specialist as, in medicine, there seems a trend; for his field will not excuse it, his patients will not permit it.

It cannot be repeated too often that sporadic experiments after a desultory course of reading, coupled, perhaps, with some superficial but high-powered instructions from equipment salesmen, will not constitute every dentist a roentgenologist; and it is pathetically true that too many dentists assume qualification upon such immature and pretended preparation. And there are publicans and sinners, these poorly trained operators, advertising charlatans, commercial roentgen-ray laboratories, who must be driven to cover, and will be when the better equipped, ethical dentists enter the field *en masse*.

This will come to pass when we reach the ideal adjustment where each clinician is his own roentgenologist. To arrive at this goal, many may find it expedient to return to their books, to attend numerous clinics, perhaps to seek close personal instruction from the experienced teachers in acclaimed schools. But brushing up on pathology, physiology, etiology, and on the modern concepts of prophylaxis, may not prove a poor policy even to the well informed. It would be a boon to the profession and public and to those whose thoroughness in such matters has grown more or less moss.

No thoughtlessly made or intended derogatory observation is this, but unvarnished truth, howsoever and whomsoever it hurts; for an appalling deficiency in the basic fundamentals of dental knowledge is too often exhibited by many with years of practice that should have been improved by continued reading. Were you to spend a few days with some active roentgenologist and hear the practitioners who come to consult him, hear their interpretations of roentgenograms and of related symptoms, hear their nervously ventured diagnoses or suggested treatments, you would find many as woefully lacking and as woefully wrong as were Dr. Tweedledum and Dr. Tweedledee to whom allusions have been made.

The alert, progressive clinician is ever searching for newer, better methods. Note the caliber of men attending the important conventions, count the outstanding dentists listening intently to valuable discussions, see the ablest of the profession observing closely the table clinics, intent on learning anything that is an improvement in theory or technique; for dentistry is certainly a progressive science, always ready to discard older ideas and substitute the tested newer thought; and a very short time will note those considered lacking who cannot interpret roentgenograms and operate the apparatus producing them.

That this shortcoming will not continue is written on the walls and in the ever-changing sands of science. In the very short future, no applicant incapable of qualifying as a roentgenologist will be licensed to practise dentistry. Some State Boards of Dental Examiners require students to make a complete full mouth roentgenographic examination of a patient and write a full report of the roentgenographic findings; and the result of that test counts no little for or against the applicant; and the theory that none lacking ability and experience to perform this routine function should be permitted to practise dentistry is so well founded that other states will follow this standard, and shortly.

Just as half-truths are often more dangerous than whole lies because more difficult to confute, in dentistry, part or half treatments may be more dangerous than none at all; for they may cover up and hide for too long a period insidious infections that might have otherwise signalled their existence earlier. The study of dentistry embraces as imperative the search for causes, the diagnosis and prognosis of the conditions besetting suspicious areas. The safe practice is to consider all areas suspicious until proven otherwise; and for this theory, the clinician as his own roentgenologist is the ideal arrangement. With the thought that competition usually results in the survival of the fittest, and recalling the philosophy that self-preservation is the first law of Nature, the older practitioners may well contemplate that the oncoming dentist will be better prepared to meet the present need of the profession in the health preservation programme of the nation in that he will be his own roentgenologist.

CHAPTER I.

THE ROENTGEN–RAY TUBE.

Following the epochal discovery of the roentgen-ray, many types of tubes were devised and tried for the purpose of producing the ray; but whatever the type, all contained gases and were extremely temperamental, for the electron supply was derived by ionization of the gases within the tubes. The tubes used by the early roentgenologists were the so-called gas tubes. Figure 2 illustrates the type of tube (a Crookes tube) with which Professor Roentgen discovered roentgen-rays.

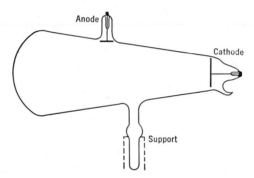

Fig. 2.—Type of tube with which Roentgen discovered x-rays.

Virtually all of the gas tubes were modifications, both in physical size and shape, of the gas tube used by Professor Roentgen. The glass bulb was pumped to a partial vacuum of about 1 mm. of mercury. The anode and cathode sealed within the tube are the terminals offering a means of passage of the high tension current through the tube. If the tube were a complete vacuum, that is, to the exclusion of all gases, there would be absolute resistance to the passage of electric current; therefore, in this type of tube, the gases present were depended upon to convey the high tension current from cathode to anode. This passage of current across the tube (from cathode to anode) is known as the cathode stream of electrons. These so-called electrons travel at such a tremendous velocity that the resulting

(32)

impact on the target of the tube causes that invisible light, roentgen-rays, to be produced.

But the gas tube, even at its best, was an uncertain factor. It had periods of "crankiness," produced by cleanup of the gas, and while it might function perfectly one day, it would be found unfit for the same purpose the next day. As a result, it could not be depended upon to operate consistently. Therefore the roentgenologist had to be equipped with a large number of gas tubes, each with its peculiar characteristic and which meant a rather large investment.

The Snook hydrogen tube was one type used quite extensively for a while. Because the amount of hydrogen within the tube could be regulated, the vacuum could be raised by removing some of the hydrogen; or, by forcing more hydrogen into the tube, the vacuum could be lowered. So the tube became known as "hard" or "soft," according to whether it was of high or low vacuum. They demanded continuous alertness of the operator to see that the proper vacuum was maintained, and a considerable amount of time was required to effect this. They have been practically discarded, since the latest modern dental equipment avoids their use.

A very important step in the progress of roentgenography was marked in 1913 when Coolidge designed a roentgen-ray tube wherein the electrons are supplied by an incandescent cathode, thereby eliminating the necessity for gas to create the electrons. These tubes are of two general kinds: the original, or universal type, and the radiator type, a later development.

The Coolidge tube differs from the early gas tubes in many ways. The glass bulb of the Coolidge tube is pumped to as high a degree of vacuum as practical to obtain. In the Coolidge tube the cathode consists of an electrically heated filament which acts as a source of electrons to bombard the target or anode. By varying the amount of current passing through the filament, the temperature of the filament can be controlled, which in turn controls the number of electrons emitted for bombarding the target, when a sufficiently high potential is placed across the cathode and anode. When using the Coolidge roentgen-ray tube, the operator has absolute control over the roentgen-ray output, and consequently techniques can be consistently and accurately reproduced. With the advent of the Coolidge hot cathode tube, the days of the erratic gas tube were over and the science of roentgenography began to make rapid strides forward.

The two Coolidge tubes used in dentistry are known as the "C.D.X. dental tube" and the "dental radiator tube." Both are

3

similar in construction, differing mainly in size and in method of radiation. Each has two terminals—the anode, or positive terminals, and the cathode, or negative terminal, both of which are sealed within a glass-walled vacuum tube.

The envelope or shell of the tube is made of lead glass, with the exception of a lime glass window which allows the useful

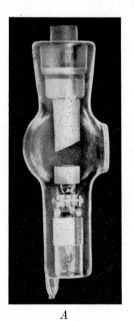

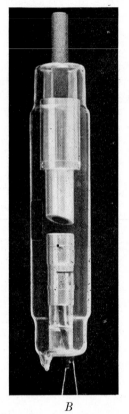

A   B

Fig. 3.—*A*, is an air-cooled type Coolidge tube as used on one type of present dental roentgen-ray equipment. *B* is a picture of the latest type oil-immersed Coolidge tube used in the dental roentgen-ray unit of the completely oil-immersed type. (General Electric *X*-ray Corp.)

roentgen-ray beam to emanate from the tube. This is a built-in protection for the operator.

The anode of practically all roentgen-ray tubes is made up of a copper bar with a tungsten button imbedded in the end, forming the target for the electron stream to hit. The angle of inclination of the face of the target is very important as it partially determines the focal spot size, which in turn determines such radiographic factors

as film detail, tube distance, speed, power required, maximum allowable film size and change in detail over the film.

In the early days of the Coolidge roentgen-ray tube, the filament
was wound in the shape of a spiral, and the face of the target was
inclined at an angle of 45 degrees to the electron stream. Such an
arrangement had several undesirable features which were chiefly
as follows:

With a 45 degree target angle and round focus electron beam, the
area on the target and the projected focal spot are about equal. By
the use of a steeper angle (20 degrees) and incorporating a rectangular stream of electrons, the projected focal spot can be made square

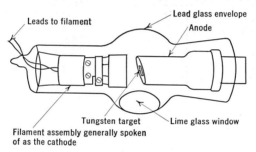

Fig. 4.—A more detailed view of the oil-immersed Coolidge roentgen-
ray tube, is made up of three parts, namely, the envelope, the anode
and the cathode. (General Electric *X*-ray Corp.)

and appreciably smaller than the area on the target. The line focus
principle is now used in the Coolidge tube.

Figure 5 shows the relation between the actual focal spot area and
the effective focal spot area in a Coolidge tube having a "line focus."
As can be seen from Figure 5, the stream of electrons bombarding
the target is rectangular in shape.

For the same effective focal spot, the area of bombardment is
much greater for the line focus tube than if a round focal spot were
used and the anode were inclined at an angle of 45 degrees instead of
20 degrees. As a result, a line focus tube can be used with a compar-
able round focus tube at the same or even higher energy rating and
with less danger of the target's being destroyed.

The physical size of a roentgen-ray tube is determined largely by
the voltage and medium under which the tube will operate. A high
voltage air-cooled tube must be designed large enough so that the
heat generated in operation will be dissipated in the surrounding

atmosphere, and in addition the tube must be long enough so that
the voltage impressed across the tube will not arc over from cathode
to anode on the outside of the envelope. The tube shown in Figure 4
is an oil-immersed tube, and consequently its physical size is relatively small, because the insulating oil in which it is immersed prevents spark-over, and at the same time is an excellent cooling agent.

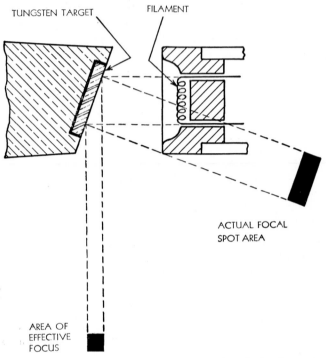

Fig. 5.—Diagram of Benson Focus, showing the relation between actual
focal spot (area of bombardment) and effective focus as projected from a
20 degree anode.   (General Electric X-ray Corp.)

CONSTRUCTION OF THE ANODE.

The anode comprises three parts: the tungsten button, or target,
the copper head in which the target is cast, and the copper stem.
(Fig. 6.)

Made of a definite grade of tungsten, determined by its degree
of crystallization, the target is treated by copper plating and

placed at the bottom of a carbon mould. On top of it is set a bar of copper, the copper having been specially treated by the addition of a chemical to assist in its melting and in the elimination of gas, and the target is then inserted into an electric vacuum furnace until the copper melts and flows around it. This operation alone takes approximately eight hours, indicating the delicacy and the precision demanded in the manufacture of these sensitive tubes.

The copper used in the stem of the anode must be of a special grade, and so rolled as to remove all cavities in the metal. Stem and head are welded together electrically, and the anode is then machined, and a fuller sleeve of dumet metal, having the same

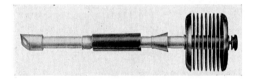

Fig. 6.—Anode of radiator type tubes; consists of tungsten button, onto which has been cast, in a vacuum, a specially purified copper head which is then electrically welded to a long copper rod which extends out through the glass of the anode arm to a copper radiator.

coefficient of expansion as glass, forms the means of making a tight seal between the glass tube and the anode. A spring-steel supporting shell is now bound on, fitting tightly into a glass anode support inside the anode arm which carries the major part of the weight of the anode and protects the glass seal.

The cathode consists of a cathode assembly or supporting structure and a tungsten filament so arranged that it can be electrically heated by a small low voltage transformer. The purpose of the tungsten filament is to provide a source of electrons to bombard the target when the filament is heated to incandescence by an electrical current.

After the filament has been heated to incandescence, it is necessary that a sufficiently high potential be placed across the anode and cathode of the roentgen-ray tube so that the electrons will be drawn from the filament to the anode with a sufficiently high velocity so that the bombardment of the target takes place and roentgen-radiation is produced.

CONSTRUCTION OF THE CATHODE.

The cathodes for all tubes are practically the same, consisting of a filament of tungsten wire supported in molybdenum parts. (Fig. 7.) Only the most carefully selected grade of tungsten can be used, for uniformity must be maintained and assured, otherwise the electron emission will vary.

In the manufacture of a cathode each process must be precisely and accurately executed, for a variation of even so little as one-thousandth of an inch from the proper dimension may make the focal spot too large or too small. The tungsten wire, cut to proper lengths, and set in a molybdenum form having a spiral groove, is placed in a hydrogen oven for some time. This insures the filament

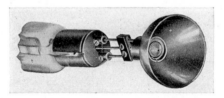

Fig. 7.—Cathode of the radiator type tube; a hemispherical metal cap surrounds the tungsten filament, to assist in the focussing.

retaining its proper form. That process completed, the filament is then bound to a slender molybdenum rod or support by a wire of tungsten, and the three are arc welded into one piece. In the cathode the filament circuit is insulated with the finest grade of India mica. The rest of the cathode is practically all molybdenum.

The filament being assembled, the free end is monel soldered to the focussing cup, the soldering being done in an atmosphere of hydrogen to prevent oxidation of the tungsten.

The assembled anode and cathode are now placed within a glass tube of selected quality and shaped to proper form, and the tube is partially exhausted and sealed. Its entire process of manufacture is predicated upon the fundamental necessity of exhausting all gases from the tube to insure an absolute vacuum.

EXHAUSTING.

The Coolidge tube gas pressure is approximately 0.05 micron—as near an absolute vacuum as has been reached. Gases are removed by pumping, a process requiring from four to five hours. But to attain the exhaustion of gases not removed in these earlier treatments, the tube is energized as in actual use, the parts being heated by overloading far beyond any temperature obtainable while using the tube as rated. There follows the testing and sealing, with a second test after a few weeks to confirm its proper functioning, before it is commercially distributed.

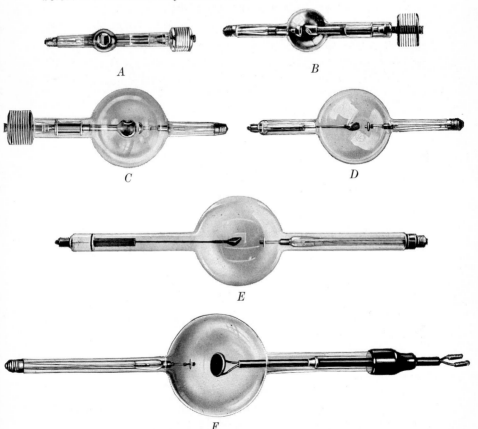

FIG. 8.—Other types of Coolidge tubes used in roentgenography and roentgenotherapy. *A*, portable radiator tube; *B*, radiator tube (for general use); *C*, 100 M.A. radiator tube; *D*, universal tube; *E*, air-cooled deep therapy tube; *F*, water-cooled deep therapy tube.

TYPES OF DENTAL TUBES.

The "dental radiator tube" is about 4 inches in diameter, with the anode and cathode at right angles to each other. A number of copper plates attached to the anode on the outside of the tube serve to radiate the tube.

The "C.D.X. dental tube" is less than 2 inches in diameter, the anode and cathode in the same plane, the heat radiation being secured by the immersion of the tube in oil. (Fig. 4.)

ELECTRON SUPPLY.

The Coolidge tube yields an electron supply that is certain and positive, which is an advantage over the uncertain and temperamental supply of the gas tube. For the source of electrons being the hot cathode filament, and the operator having control of the number of available electrons simply by changing the filament current, the increase or decrease of the electrons given off is merely a matter of increasing or decreasing the heat of the filament.

PRODUCTION OF THE ROENTGEN-RAY.

Electrical circuits used in dental roentgen-ray equipment can be broken down into three major divisions, namely, the roentgen-ray tube, the high voltage circuit, and the control circuit. Each of these divisions plays an equally important part in the operation of the unit, because without any one, the unit as a whole will not operate. It must be kept in mind, however, that just mere combinations of tubes, high tension transformers, and control circuits will not necessarily result in the production of a high quality roentgenogram. Therefore, in selecting these various combinations, they must be so chosen that the finished unit will be conveniently practical, highly efficient, and 100 per cent electrically safe, and last, but not least, manufactured by an organization having experience, facilities, and integrity.

The roentgen-ray tube is considered the heart of any roentgen-ray unit. The function of the tube is to produce roentgen-radiation which is electro-magnetic radiation of very short wave length, generated by the bombardment of a target (usually tungsten) with a relatively high velocity stream of electrons.

The ordinary light ray, as we all know, does not have the power to penetrate opaque substances. The roentgen-ray does have that power, however, and therefore reveals to us many things which would otherwise be invisible to the eye. Roentgen-rays themselves are not visible, but their properties of affecting photographic emulsions and fluorescent screens (deposits of barium platinocyanide crystals or calcium tungstate crystals on cardboard) renders the results of the passage of roentgen-rays through a substance visible to the eye.

Roentgen-rays are produced by the passage of a high-tension electric current through a glass-walled vacuum tube. The current results from the projection of minute electric particles (electrons) from the one metal terminal, the cathode, to the anode or target, the other metal terminal, the roentgen-rays originating at the point of impact of the electrons on the target and travelling from that point in all directions, except where dense materials obstruct or prevent their passage. Where passing through bodies of varied density, a portion of the rays entering the denser areas are absorbed.

Investigations show these rays to be identical in their nature with light and electric waves, though of wave lengths shorter than the shortest light waves, and as the roentgen-rays travel in straight lines, into, through, and out of material bodies, they cannot be deflected by mirrors or lenses for the purpose of optical focus or concentration as can be done with light.

Being invisible, the presence of the roentgen-rays is determined only by some of the effects they produce when acting on material bodies, as:

(*a*) Effect on the emulsion of a photographic plate.
(*b*) Excitation of light on certain crystals (fluorescence).
(*c*) Stimulative or destructive action on living cells.

ELECTRONS.

The modern concept of atoms involves the idea of their general electrical constitution. From any atom there may be abstracted one or more small negative charges, all precisely alike, whose properties are in no wise dependent upon the atom from which they come, and all are capable of existence by themselves without the presence of the remainder of the atom. These little bodies have been named electric ions, or electrons. An electron is able to respond to electric force and to acquire velocity under such force. When in motion they show all the characteristics of an electric current. Electrons have extremely small mass and volume and may acquire extreme velocity.

The radio-active breakdown of atoms results in a sudden acquisition of electronic velocity, producing gamma rays—the primary form of the roentgen-ray. In the roentgen-ray tubes the high-speed electron is stopped in its flight by the interposition of the target, a loss of velocity ensuing, and this sudden change in the velocity of the electrons causes the origin of the roentgen-ray. The problem of the ray production resolves itself into:

1. Separation of electrons from atoms. In the Coolidge tube the electrons are set free from the atoms contained in the tungsten filament by the action of heat.

2. Giving them high speed. To secure high speed high voltage must be available.

3. Concentrating them on a small area. The electrons must be urged toward a small area in order to assure concentration of the cathode stream on the focal spot of the anode.

4. Stopping them with sufficient suddenness. Due to the great rise in temperature at the point of electron concentration, only metals of high melting-point can be employed as a barrier. Tungsten is most commonly used.

Outflow of Radiation, Time-distance Relation.—As radiation spreads out from the focal spot on the target, the amount or intensity of radiation received in a given time on any fixed area decreases when the distance of the receiving surface from the focal spot is increased. This decrease always follows the inverse square law. Thus, if four arbitrary units reach a given area at 10 inches from the target, the same area 20 inches from the target will only get one-fourth as much radiation in the same time, *i. e.*, 1 unit. Therefore, in order to get the same radiation to this area at the increased distance, the time must be increased as the square of the distance. Thus, if at 10 inches, two seconds are required, at 20 inches $2 \times \left(\dfrac{20}{10}\right)^2$ seconds, or eight seconds, will be required.

Amount of Radiation.—For our purpose the photographic measure of roentgen-ray radiation is sufficiently accurate, and determines the usefulness of the rays in practice.

Quality.—Quality determines the ability of the rays to pass through flesh and bone. It depends on the voltage used to drive the current across the space between cathode and anode, and is best expressed in terms of voltage. Current passing through a tube is of no value unless the voltage used is able to break down from 2 to 6 inches of air between the points of the spark-gap. The relation of voltage requirement to the length of the spark-gap in inches is approximately ten times the gap in inches + 10,000 volts. Thus a 3-inch gap requires $3 \times 10,000$ volts + 10,000 volts = 40,000 volts.

Penetration.—The most characteristic feature of the roentgen-rays is their ability to pass through material quite opaque to other types of radiation. In all cases there is some absorption, but the amount left after passing through any layer of material varies according to the composition of the roentgen-ray beam.

ELEMENTARY TERMINOLOGY.

The electrical terms used most frequently in connection with roentgenography are as follows:

Volt.—The unit of electric motive force. It is the unit in which is measured the tendency of a charge to move from one place to another.

Current.—A measure of the number of electrons passing a given point on a conductor per second.

Ampère.—The unit of electric current, or the amount of electric current. Amperage is the most dangerous part of electricity.

Ohm.—The unit of electric resistance.

Resistance.—Any objection offered to the passage of an electric current by material included in the circuit.

Power.—The ability of the electric current to do work.

Watt.—The unit of electrical power. It is the power of a current of 1 ampère in a region where it loses 1 volt.

Ohm's Law.—The strength of the electric current equals the pressure divided by the resistance:

$$\text{Ampères} = \frac{\text{Volts}}{\text{Ohms}}$$

$$\text{Volts} = \text{Ampères} \times \text{Ohms}$$

$$\text{Ohms} = \frac{\text{Volts}}{\text{Ampères}}$$

1 kilovolt equals 1000 volts.

1 milliampère equals $\frac{1}{1000}$ of an ampère.

1 kilowatt equals 1000 watts.

Kilowatt Hour.—One kilowatt maintained for one hour.

KINDS OF ELECTRIC CURRENT USED.

Two kinds of electric current used or supplied by the modern power plants are the "direct" current and the "alternating" current.

In the direct current, called D.C. in the electrical world, the electron flow is in only one direction; while in the alternating current, called A.C., the electron flow is first in one direction for a short time and then the flow decreases and a reverse flow occurs.

ROENTGEN–RAY CURRENT–VOLTAGE REQUIREMENTS.

The modern dental equipment used for the production of the roentgen-ray requires a current of 10 milliampères and a voltage of 40,000. As this high-voltage requirement cannot be met by a generator, the necessary voltage is secured by the use of a transformer. Until Snook (1908) introduced the first high-tension transformer, the induction coil was used. But the transformer has approximately twice the efficiency of the induction coil.

The Roentgen-ray Transformer.—The function of the high tension transformer is to produce the necessary potential for the proper operation of the roentgen-ray tube. Such a transformer should be so designed that it will withstand the duties imposed upon it by high voltage operation over a long period of time.

To give the reader a physical picture of what a high tension transformer does, let us consider a roentgen-ray unit in operation. Suppose that for proper operation a roentgen-ray tube requires 55,000 volts. The line voltage in most dental offices is 110 volts; hence the function of the high tension transformer is to step this 110 volts up to 55,000 volts. Disregarding all electrical losses, suppose a transformer were designed so that for every one turn on the primary side there were 500 turns on the secondary side. This would give a transformation ratio of 1 to 500, and if 110 volts were impressed across the primary side, the voltage across the secondary side would be 55,000 volts. For more detailed information, see Figure 10.

The voltage of a high tension transformer is dangerously high, and it would be sometimes fatal for an operator or patient to come in contact with any part of the high tension system. The earlier types of dental roentgen-ray units on the market had an exposed tube and high tension system which made them most dangerous and awkward to operate. However, practically all the later types of dental roentgen-ray equipment on the market today are so designed that they are 100 per cent electrically safe.

The use of a transformer to increase voltage involves two distinct circuits: one, known as the primary circuit, and connected through a control device known as an auto-transformer to the supply line or generator; the other, known as the secondary circuit, insulated from the primary and connected to the tube terminals.

The transformer changes voltage approximately in the ratio of the number of turns in the primary circuit to the number of turns in the secondary circuit, and loses amperage in inverse ratio. Thus, if a transformer has 500 turns in the secondary to 1 turn in the primary, the secondary voltage would be 500 times the voltage of the primary, and the secondary amperage $\frac{1}{500}$ of the amperage of the primary.

The characteristics of the primary circuit are: relative low voltage; carries a current of variable ampères; is reasonably safe to touch; requires good metallic contact at all connections.

The characteristics of the secondary circuit are: high voltage; small wire; carries a current of only milliampères; relatively dangerous to touch; will pass current across loose connections or even through some insulating material.

Auto-transformer.—Most dental roentgen-ray units are equipped with what is known as a voltage compensator. This device enables the operator to adjust his unit to the proper voltage from the line on which he operates immediately prior to the exposure. It is a manual control and has a very definite place on every unit. This is used as a control device to reduce the line voltage to that which is applied to the primary circuit of the transformer. It is a step-down transformer, having fewer turns in the secondary circuit than in the primary, and consists of a continuous coil of wire wound around an iron core, with taps passing out to the control buttons. If alternating current be supplied to any particular segment of such a coil, a voltage will be induced in that part of the winding bearing the same relation to the applied voltage that the number of turns of this part of the winding bears to the number of turns in the whole coil. The action depends upon self-induction in a single coil rather than on mutual induction between two coils.

Stabilization.—The function of the control circuit is to give the operator some control over his roentgen-ray equipment, thereby allowing him to duplicate techniques and thus have a standard technique to follow. Too many controls or variables on a unit are as bad if not worse than not enough controls on the equipment, because the former tend to make radiography complicated, resulting in a poor end result. Certain controls on roentgen-ray equipment are preferable to other controls because of the fact that they affect the end results more.

The operating voltage of a roentgen-ray unit determines its penetration and the milliamperage passing through the tube determines the density of the part being radiographed on the film. In most localities, the line voltage does not fluctuate more than 5 per cent; therefore, it would be preferable to have some control over the current passing through the tube than to have control over the voltage energizing the high tension transformer. If there is a fluctuation of 5 per cent in the line voltage, the milliamperage passing through the roentgen-ray tube will vary approximately 100 per cent from the miniumum required for the roentgenogram, unless there is a stabilizer in the tube circuit which will maintain the current at a constant value. If there is a 15 per cent change in line voltage without a stabilizer in the circuit, the milliamperage will vary in excess of 200 per cent of the minimum.

Keeping these figures in mind, suppose that someone in the same building turned on a sterilizer or motor while the roentgen-ray unit was being used. This load thrown upon the line would cause the voltage to drop, which in turn would cause a decrease in milliamperage passing through the tube, which in turn would cause the resulting roentgenogram to be too light. Now, by having a stabilizer in the tube circuit, this condition could not exist because the current passing through the tube would be maintained automatically at a constant value, provided the voltage drop was not in excess of 15 per cent. The stabilizer also works if the voltage is suddenly increased on the line, except that in this case, the stabilizer not only prevents the roentgenogram from being too dark, but it also protects the tube from an excessive current which might destroy it. Probably the most universally used stabilizer of this type on the market today is the Kearsley Stabilizer.

There is one other type of stabilizer used for regulating the tube current which is known as the Universal type stabilizer. This type of stabilizer automatically regulates the voltage, which in turn regulates the current passing through the tube.

It is interesting to analyze the action of the Kearsley Stabilizer in the tube circuit. Figure 9 is a schematic drawing of the Kearsley Stabilizer with the various parts lettered.

Lead M of the stabilizer is connected to the cathode side of the roentgen-ray tube. Lead N is connected to the primary side of the filament transformer. The current passing through the roentgen-ray tube must pass through the solenoid marked A. When the current passing through the tube exceeds a certain predetermined value, the magnetic field set up by the solenoid is great enough to pull the movable contact B away from the fixed contact C, thus causing the resistance D to be inserted in the circuit. With resistance D in the circuit, the current passing through the filament transformer is reduced, which in turn reduces the temperature of the filament in the roentgen-ray tube, and consequently less current passes through the tube. The movable contact B of the stabilizer is connected with a spring which opposes the action of the solenoid A, and consequently this movable contact B constantly vibrates when the roentgen-ray tube is energized. Suppose that the current through the roentgen-ray tube suddenly decreased in value? The tension of spring E is greater than the force of the solenoid A, and consequently movable contact B is held against C, thereby shorting our resistance D which causes a greater amount of current to flow through the filament transformer, thus causing an increase in temperature of the filament in the roentgen-ray tube, which, in turn, causes the flow of current through the tube to increase until it has reached its

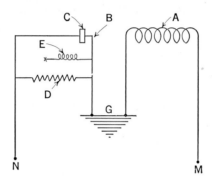

Fig. 9.—Kearsley stabilizer. *A*, solenoid; *B*, movable contact; *C*, fixed contact; *D*, resistance; *E*, spring; *G*, common terminal; *M*, terminal connected to cathode; *N*, terminal connected to filament transformer primary.

normal value. When the current exceeds its normal value, the stabilizer will again act to decrease the amount of current passing through the tube, and thus restore the balance. The foregoing picture will give the reader some idea of how the Kearsley stabilizer is constantly working to maintain an even current passing through the roentgen-ray tube.

The Coolidge Filament Transformer.—This is simply a step-down transformer which reduces the line voltage of 110 volts to one of 12 volts, which heats the tungsten filament in the Coolidge tube, and the filament in turn gives off the electrons.

Rotary Converters.—The roentgen-ray transformer will operate only when its primary circuit is supplied with alternating current.

So when the source of supply is a direct current, a rotary converter must be used to change the direct current to an alternating current. It is practically a motor generator, the D.C. current passing into the motor on one side and coming out on the other side as an A.C. current. There is, however, approximately a loss of 30 per cent of the line voltage during this operation. Thus, a converter operating on 110 volts D.C. will deliver only 77 volts A.C. In view of the fact that the voltage output of any transformer is controlled by the ratio of the turns of the primary and secondary windings, respectively, it is immaterial with a properly designed roentgen-ray transformer whether the transformer is energized with 77 volt or 110 volt current and the penetrability of the roentgen-rays is the same in either instance. Where the 77 volt current is used for energizing the primary, the number of turns on the primary winding is less than is necessary where the 110 volt current is used.

Timers.—The timer of a roentgen-ray unit is a very important part of the control circuit. The exposure timer serves not only to automatically measure the correct radiographic exposure time, but also to control the current to both the high tension transformer and the tube filament transformer. To insure accuracy, the speed of the timing mechanism is controlled by magnetic dampening through a disk which revolves between poles of a permanent magnet. This principle is similar to that used in electric meters for measuring watt-hour consumption, where accuracy and dependability are first essentials.

The component parts of a roentgen-ray unit have been discussed. Now let us consider a roentgen-ray unit in its entirety. The following diagrams are given with the idea in mind of bringing out some of the outstanding improvements in the dental roentgen-ray circuit up to the present time.

Figure 10 is a wiring diagram of an early type roentgen-ray circuit, using a right angle type Coolidge roentgen-ray tube. This circuit has the barest essentials necessary for operating the Coolidge roentgen-ray tube. There were many undesirable features about this circuit which made it objectionable to operate. The tube and high tension wires were exposed, and consequently if the operator or patient came in contact with them, they were in danger of being severely shocked. There was no timer incorporated in this circuit, and consequently the exposure time was left entirely to the judgment of the operator, which was usually quite a variable factor. In general, it might be said that the operator had absolutely no control over the circuit whatsoever.

In order to give the operator some control of the roentgen-ray unit so that techniques could be duplicated without a great deal of difficulty, it was deemed advisable to incorporate a timer in the circuit so that the exposure could be accurately timed and terminated at the end of a specified interval. In addition, a voltage compensator was added so that slight changes in voltages could be compensated before exposure was started.

Figure 11 is a wiring diagram of this improved circuit with the additions shown by heavier lines and bold type. However, the

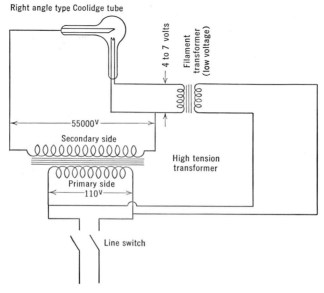

Fɪɢ. 10.

circuit shown in Figure 11 still retains many of the disadvantages of the circuit shown in Figure 10, namely, relatively dangerous to both operator and patient, awkward to handle which in turn made dental radiography unnecessarily difficult, and it still lacked the refinement of control that was desired.

In an effort to improve upon the dental roentgen-ray unit, Dr. W. D. Coolidge, in 1920, conceived the idea that if a unit were so constructed that the high tension transformer, roentgen-ray tube, and filament transformer were immersed in oil in a single grounded container, then the roentgen-ray unit would be 100 per cent electrically

4

safe, and the danger of high voltage would be removed once and for all. With this idea in mind, Dr. Coolidge proceeded to make some very radical changes in the design of roentgen-ray equipment, and in September, 1921, presented and described the first shockproof and 100 per cent electrically safe dental roentgen-ray unit to the American Roentgen Society. His basic conception proved very successful.

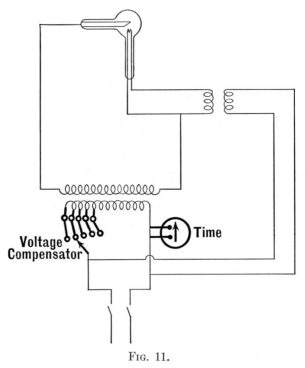

Fig. 11.

Since Dr. Coolidge's announcement in 1921, there have been developed three basic types of shockproof roentgen-ray units on the market, namely the shockproof cable type high tension fed systems, air-cooled shielded type systems, and the completely oil-immersed high tension transformer and Coolidge roentgen-ray tube.

The air-cooled shielded type roentgen-ray unit (Fig. 12) is very efficient. The tube, roentgen-ray protected by a lead shield, is placed in an air circulating chamber of the shockproof head separated from the oil immersed transformer. The center of the high tension system, grounded to provide safety, is equipped with the new Coolidge line focus tube, which is protected against any possible overloads by the use of a circuit breaker. Figures 12 and 27, 13 and 23 are cutaway sections showing an air-cooled shielded type roentgen-ray unit and a completely oil-immersed roentgen-ray unit.

Figure 13 is a cutaway section of a Coolidge dental roentgen-ray unit showing how the high tension transformer, filament transformer

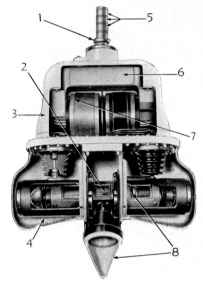

Fig. 12.—1, Full circumference, steel bearing; 2, straight line target of tube; 3, roentgen-ray head; 4, air cooling chamber providing for highest tube efficiency requirements; 5, contact rings form electrical connections with double spring wiper contacts; 6, oil immersed transformer; 7, transformer; 8, tube and focusing cone move simultaneously. (Courtesy of Ritter Dental Co.)

and Coolidge roentgen-ray tube are immersed in oil in one single container, thus rendering the roentgen-ray unit completely 100 per cent electrically safe. Such a design has many advantages besides the fact that it is absolutely shockproof. Some of these are humidity-proof, altitude-proof, better cooling conditions, tamper-proof, and many others. In order to take care of changes in oil volume due to ambient temperature, a bellows was mounted in the unit so that when the oil expanded, the bellows would contract, thus taking care of the increased volume, or expand when the temperature decreased, thus taking care of a decrease in oil volume. A Kearsley stabilizer as described in Figure 5 is incorporated in the tube circuit so that a constant milliamperage is maintained at all times when an exposure is being made.

In order to give the reader a more thorough picture, Figure 14 is a wiring diagram of the oil-immersed roentgen-ray unit shown in

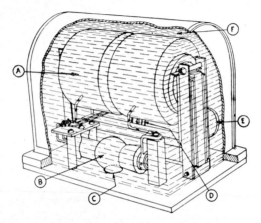

Fig. 13.—Showing how the C.D.X. Coolidge tube, high tension transformer and filament transformer are completely immersed in oil in one container. (*A*) High tension transformer; (*B*) Coolidge tube; (*C*) lime glass window of tube; (*D*) filament transformer; (*E*) oil expansion chamber; (*F*) oil-filled container. (General Electric *X*-ray Corp.)

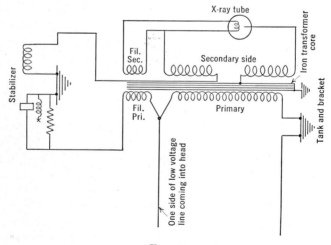

Fig. 14.

Figures 13 and 23. As shown by the wiring diagram, the high tension system and Coolidge tube is completely sealed away so that there is not any chance of the operator or patient coming in contact with it. There is one low voltage lead (which is completely insulated) that runs from the voltage compensator to the head. The bracket and tank form the second or return lead, which is similar to the rail return on a street-car line.

The idea of oil immersion of the tube as well as the winding in a single container has proved so successful that at the present writing deep therapy units of 400,000 volts are being manufactured with their high tension system and Coolidge roentgen-ray tube completely oil-immersed.

CHAPTER II.

ROENTGEN–RAY DERMATOSIS.

One part of the history of roentgenography will never be told. That part is the number of minor casualties following the wake of inexperienced or careless operators. Too many are prone to hold lightly the thoughtless handling of the delicately dangerous apparatus, dangerous both to the patient and the operator—if not manipulated perfectly and delicately as the instrument demands it to be handled.

A roentgen-ray burn, to use the simpler terminology, is an insidious danger; for it may not be known or felt to have left its mark until many successive burns have brought about a chronic condition that will require careful nursing to combat.

Every possible precaution for protection against the acknowledged deleterious action of the rays should be followed. The effect of the roentgen-rays are cumulative in their action: the small amount of radiation received today is added to the amount received yesterday, and so on until the tissues have received an intolerable amount of radiation that produces an erythema.

Throughout the entire first years of the use of the roentgen-ray the pioneer operators were subjecting themselves to the most hazardous dangers. They knew little and thought less about the danger until attention to the hazards incident to exposure to the roentgen-ray was first called by Marcuse,[1] "The production of an alopecia and a dermatitis resembling sunburn."

Roentgen-ray dermatitis in its incipient state manifests itself in somewhat the same way as ordinary sunburn. There is a slight discoloration, the skin becomes dry, and often is accompanied by a tingling and burning sensation. A continued exposure to the rays, however, will produce a chronic roentgen-ray dermatosis, the symptoms of which are seen especially on the uncovered parts of the operator. The picture is clear and should never be difficult to diagnose: the skin has a harsh, dry feel, and scattered over its surface are brownish, macular areas of pigmentation. Telangiectases are also to be seen to a greater or less degree. In places the skin may appear lardaceous, shiny, hard, thickened and bound

---

[1] Marcuse: Deutsch. med. Wchnschr., 1896.

down, as it were, to the bones, and stretched as if it were too small to cover the parts affected. This condition is seen mostly in the hands, as the hands are more exposed to the deleterious action of the rays. The nails are friable, with broken-off ends, and longitudinal fissures over their surface. In addition, there is a piling up of the nail tissues under the friable, free distal ends. The skin around the nails is also affected with a piling-up of epidermis and the formation of hang-nails. In fact, the presence of hang-nails and of dry skin on the hands is usually the first precursor of a chronic roentgen-ray dermatitis.

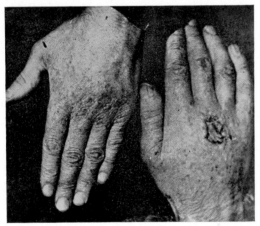

FIG. 15.—Advanced chronic radiodermatitis on the backs of hands. (Cole.)

If the dermatitis is more advanced the presence of keratoses is noticed over the surfaces of the hands, and cracks appear especially over the dorsum of the knuckles and finger-joints. Some of these may even break down, and one may note ulcerations, indolent in type. Perhaps some of these have healed over, and then there are keratoses, cracks, scales, ulcers and healed scars scattered here and there over the dorsum of the hands and even of the face. (Fig. 15.)

Some of the ulcers may refuse to heal, and some of the keratoses may increase in size, degenerate and become malignant, showing ultimately the clinical characteristics of epitheliomas. As a rule, however, this condition becomes manifest later, but all authorities warn us that generally it is impossible to make an early diagnosis of malignant change except through the use of the microscope. In advanced cases one may find ten, fifteen, twenty or more areas of malignant change on the hands of a single patient. If we wait for gross changes it may be too late.

Hesse[1] collected records of 94 cases of roentgen-ray dermatosis with malignant change, 54 of which occurred in physicians or technicians. In this list sarcoma had been diagnosed once; either sarcoma or carcinoma, three times; and carcinoma in the remainder. The time elapsing from the first use of the roentgen-ray to the malignancy was from four to fourteen years, with a median of 37 cases of nine years. The time from the first dermatitis to the first

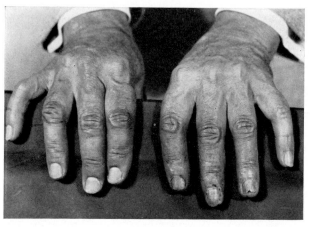

Fig. 16.—A photograph of a Philadelphia dentist's hands, who for a number of years, took roentgenograms of his patient's teeth holding the film with one of his hands in the patient's mouth while the exposure was being made. The one which he employed in that fashion, shows a characteristic and well-marked roentgen dermatitis. In this day and age this condition is inexcusable, and shows an absolute ignorance, and carelessness on the part of the operator. Note the condition of the nails and fingers of the left hand. (Courtesy of Dr. I. Robert Andrews.)

malignancy varied from one to eleven years, being four and a half years in 20 cases. But these figures, you will note, are merely from the reported cases, and there is every reason to suspect that dangerous results have been found under a much less elapsed time of exposure to the rays.

Alopecia, loss of the hair, often results from too long or too often repeated exposures to the roentgen-ray. But, except in

[1] Hesse: Fortschr. a. d. Geb. d. Roentgenstrahlen, **7**, 82–92, 1911.

extreme exposures, in many cases the loss of the hair is not always permanent. (Fig. 18.) This thought, however, must not lessen vigilant caution of the operator.

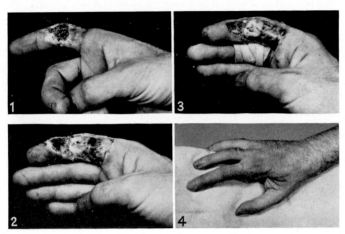

FIG. 17.—Hyperkeratosis of right index finger that increased progressively to extend from the distal interphalangeal joint to the base of the index finger on the palmar surface ultimately requiring removal of the entire diseased area by amputation. (Courtesy of Dr. George E. Pfahler.)

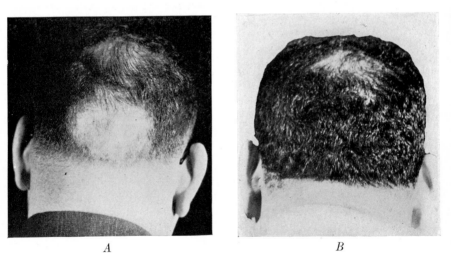

FIG. 18.—*A*, Alopecia. Produced by too much radiation. *B*, same case as shown in *A*, six months later, hair having been restored. However, too much radiation causes a permanent loss of the hair.

Course of Events in Chronic Roentgen-ray Dermatoses.—Constant exposure to the roentgen-rays causes a series of degenerative changes in the skin. Pilosebaceous and sweat glands are affected very early, creating dryness of the skin and a loss of hair. Thereafter comes a gradual change in the corium due to the effect on the blood supply of the parts exposed. An obliterating endarteritis results, and with it an hyaline collagenous change in and a thickening of the corium occurs. This leads to that hard, lardaceous, bound down appearance commonly seen in such cases. The corium seems to become more affected than the epidermis and degenerates especially in an area just under the epidermis.

Nature attempts to overcome this starving of the tissues through newly formed capillaries and the opening up of capillaries already present. The epidermis, no longer able to get its normal blood supply from the usual sources, reacts in quite a typical manner. It sets out to find a new blood supply, sending down long epidermal processes toward the weakened upper layers of the dermis. The epidermal cells multiply more and more rapidly in their search for blood, and more mitoses are seen. If a fissure appears in the corium as a result of an area of degeneration from lack of capillary supply, as from a sclerosed vessel, the epidermis steps in to fill the gap. If the gap is too large to fill, or if a severe secondary infection intervenes, an ulcer forms; and in old ulcers and keratoses, the epidermal cells finally become almost parasitic; growing wild and invading the corium— a true epidermoid carcinoma on top of a chronic roentgen-ray dermatosis.

Treatment.—In the treatment of chronic roentgen-ray dermatitis, the use of the quartz-lamp therapy, carbon dioxide snow, electrocoagulation, surgery, and in some cases radium and roentgen-ray treatment is indicated. But the best treatment for all types of roentgen-ray dermatitis is prophylaxis, or the prevention of the disease. One should protect himself from unnecessary exposure.

In the acute stages of roentgen-ray dermatitis the best results are obtained by using astringent lotions, such as Dodd's solution (phenol, 1.85 parts; zinc oxide, 15.5 parts; glycerin, 4 parts; lime water, sufficient to make 250 parts); or hychlorite solution, 1 to 20 or 1 to 30 in water, is of value. Cole[1] finds glycerite of tannic acid, 25 per cent, in hammamelis water, to be a very soothing lotion. It is applied frequently and allowed to dry on the affected parts.

---

[1] Cole: Chronic Roentgen-ray Dermatosis as Seen in the Professional Man, Jour. Am. Med. Assn., vol. **84**, No. 12, p. 365.

The *erythema dose* of the roentgen-ray at a target-plate distance of 10 inches may be said to be twelve hundred milliampère-seconds. By multiplying the number of milliampères used by the time of exposure in seconds we obtain the exposure-time in milliampère-seconds. The result is then divided into twelve hundred milliampère-seconds which will give us the number of exposures we may make. For example:

10 ma. × 5 seconds = 50 ma.-seconds.

1200 ma.-seconds ÷ 50 ma.-seconds = 24, or the number of exposures that may be made without unduly exposing the subject beyond the danger line. But upon even approaching the erythema dose, a period of three weeks should elapse before the patient is again subjected to any radiation.

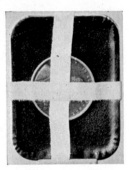

FIG. 19. — Penny placed upon a film, which is carried to test for radiation.

Idiosyncrasy.—There are individuals who are more susceptible to the rays than others. And while these may be the exceptions to the rule, alertness must be ever the watchword of the operator in all cases. Two interesting cases of this type were represented by females, each about thirty years of age, who received an erythema after an exposure of fifty milliampère-seconds. But upon investigation it was found that both patients would receive a sunburn at the seashore in the middle of the winter. In cases such as these it is best to refrain from any avoidable radiation.

Radiation Test.—The operator may determine whether he is subjecting himself to exposure by placing a penny on the emulsion side of a small dental film packet, keeping it in place with straps of adhesive tape. (Fig. 19.) The packet is them placed in the vest pocket with the emulsion side of the film facing the tube. This is carried in the pocket for a period of two weeks, at the end of which it is taken into the dark room and developed. A control, used in the form of a film which has not been subjected to the action of the rays, is developed at the same time. If an image or outline of the penny appears on the film so carried in the pocket, it is conclusive evidence that the operator is receiving radiation and should immediately take the necessary measures to protect himself. (Fig. 20.)

Ample protection may be obtained by placing a screen covered with a sheet of lead $\frac{1}{8}$ inch in thickness between the operator and the tube. The screen should be at least 2 feet wide and 6 feet high.

The operator should never stand in the hemisphere of activity. The rays start from a point on the anode and pass out in all directions. While the modern tubes are covered with a lead glass (Fig. 21) which prevents the escape of the majority of the rays, yet there is an opening in the lead-glass shield opposite the anode for the direct rays to pass out, and this opening becomes most dangerous. The rays form a cone, the focal spot being the apex of the cone and the opening in the lead-glass shield being the base at that point, but as the rays go beyond this region the base of the cone

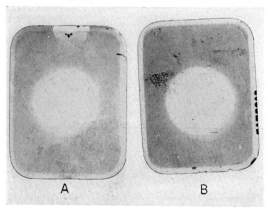

Fig. 20.—*A*, Outline of penny on film after one week's trial. *B*, outline of penny after a period of two weeks, showing more pronounced exposure.

becomes larger as the distance is increased. (Fig. 22.) Therefore often the inexperienced operator or the one who believes the propaganda that the small dental units are absolutely safe may expose himself to too much radiation and later suffer dire results.

The operator should never hold the film in the mouth for a patient, nor should he allow his assistant to do it; for once this practice is begun, it is quite thoughtlessly repeated, leading toward the danger line before its effects are noticed. (Fig. 16.)

DENTAL FLUOROSCOPY.

Though discussed briefly, it is not with the intent of dismissing abruptly the topic of fluoroscopic examinations of the teeth and surrounding structures. Whatever satisfactory experience has resulted from the technique is a gain for dentistry, but the essential question in any scientific procedure is the point of its superiority over other methods in gaining its objective, and when contemplating the several factors incident to a method under consideration, we must consider

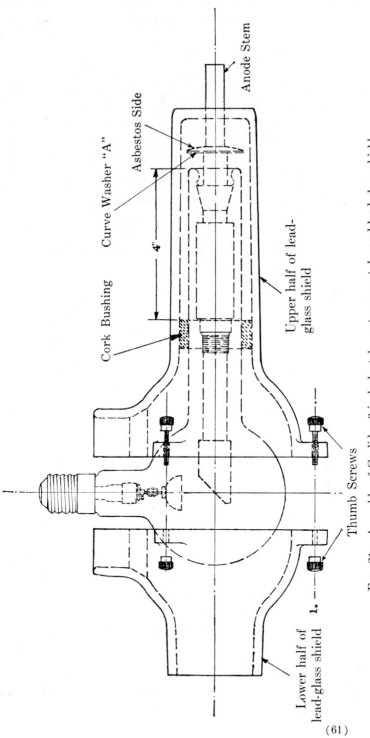

Anode Stem

Asbestos Side

Curve Washer "A"

4"

Cork Bushing

Upper half of lead-
glass shield

Thumb Screws

Lower half of
lead-glass shield

1.

Fig. 21.—Assembly of Coolidge 3-inch dental roentgen-ray tube and lead-glass shield.

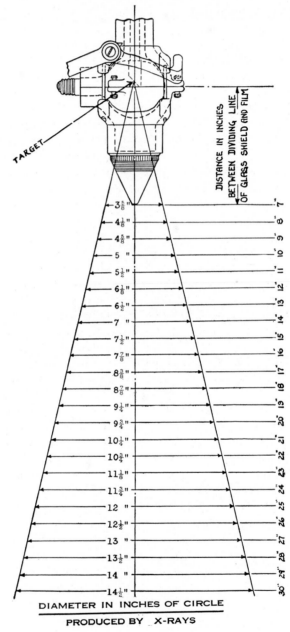

DIAMETER IN INCHES OF CIRCLE

PRODUCED BY X-RAYS

Fig. 22.—Demonstrating the cone of rays being emitted from the target, the base of the cone becoming greater as the distance is increased; the operator's body should never be within this area.

the convenience, the danger, the time, the cost, always conceding the talent of the operator.

Both roentgenology and fluoroscopy aiming with the same purpose in dentistry, the primary requirement for dental diagnosis is the sharpness of detail we do disclose in the roentgenogram, a sharpness of detail probably greater than is required for many other parts of the body. The fine distinctions in densities necessary to a dentist must appear with the least possible doubt, for many small areas are met with such slight differences in density that to distinguish these differences is difficult; even the slightest variation in density of the tissues surrounding the teeth and of the bone are important guides on which the dentist relies for his diagnosis, and roentgenographic examinations have proven the most accurate and trustworthy method of depicting these variations.

The fluoroscope precludes showing the detail sharpness dentistry demands. Even in fluoroscoping a part of the body as thin as the hand, the resulting detail on the fluoroscopic screen is inferior to that produced roentgenographically. So it must be deemed inferior from the diagnostic standpoint. Then there is the point of proper angulation so important in dental roentgenology; and that part of the technique certainly cannot be disregarded in dental fluoroscopy; but it is difficult to determine accurately the angles being employed during the fluoroscopic examination.

Because radiation mounts rapidly during fluoroscopic examinations they must be conducted with greater care as to skin tolerance. Even under the most favorable conditions, a patient will receive more radiation during a fluoroscopic examination than he would receive during a roentgenologic examination. This is likewise true of the operator.

The danger to the operator should not be overlooked. However carefully used, dental fluoroscopy brings him into the plane of radiation too often for safety. If we but contemplate a fluoroscopic examination of the maxillary molars, whatever the type of fluoroscope employed, the difficulty of avoiding the radiation angulated to penetrate the anatomical structures surrounding them while attempting to observe ocularly the condition disclosed may be perceived. Nor can we overlook the truth that the effect of the roentgen-rays on the skin varies directly according to the length of exposure: an exposure of one second at 10 milliampères would have twice the effect upon the skin that would result from a similar exposure at 5 milliampères. Whatever the dosage, whatever time exposed, there is seemingly a greater vulnerability offered by the operator using the fluoroscope than by using the roentgenogram.

It takes considerable time to accommodate the eyes for them, and the dental office necessarily being well lighted, the dentist would require ten or more minutes accommodating his eyes to the darkened room before attempting them, so the total time taken in a fluoroscopic examination would usually exceed that required for dental roentgenology.

OSTEORADIONECROSIS.

Osteoradionecrosis is a frequent complication in the treatment of cancer of the oral cavity by irradiation; and it is so striking, and often so rapid and explosive in its onset and so serious in its resultant morbidity and mortality, that it is the great responsibility of the dentist to recognize its faintest appearance.

To understand the reaction of bone to irradiation we must know the peculiar gross and histological architecture of bone tissue: that bone cells derive from osteoblasts which have become enclosed in a bone space or lacuna; that the bone cells connect one with the other, receiving nourishment through very fine processes known as canaliculi; that the outer surface of the bone receives a large portion of its nourishment from the periosteal blood-vessels entering its substance through Volkmann's canals; that the blood-vessels of the Haversian canals and the nutrient artery supply the deeper portions of the bone and the marrow. This blood system forms a rich and delicate vascular network enclosed in a rigid frame of bone tissue, a structure highly vulnerable to the effect of irradiation.

Ewing[1] found the periosteum very susceptible to irradiation, gross swelling and thickening occurring and the periosteum stripping easily from the bone after sizeable therapeutic doses. An histological examination shows the inner surface of the periosteum presenting a thick hyaline layer without cells; and the layer of osteoblasts usually found on the inner surface of the periosteum in contact with the bone may be absent. This explains the lack of bone regeneration after sequestrectomy or subperiosteal jaw resection: The arterioles probably strangulated by a postirradiation swelling of all the coats comprising the walls of the blood-vessels.

Following irradiation the bone often shows osteoporosis, the trabeculæ becoming narrowed and irregular, the volume of fatty marrow increased; the bony structure is less substantial and extensive obliterative sclerosis of the nutrient vessels occurs.

The possibilities for osteoradionecrosis developing seem fairly

---

[1] Ewing, J.: Tissue Reactions to Radiation, Am. Jour. Roentgenol. and Rad. Therapy, **15**, 93–115, 1926.

obvious when we realize the patients are probably well past middle age, a stage when a certain amount of osteoporosis is fairly common and the appearance of arteriosclerosis of the vascular structures of the bone are not unexpected. Before treatment is begun, even, there is frequently a deplorable intraoral condition due to neglect of ordinary hygienic measures. Of 170 patients in whom satisfactory data pertaining to the teeth were obtained, Watson and Scarborough[1] report only 7 showed teeth in good condition; 27 had fair teeth, 100 had poor teeth, and 36 were edentulous. Such patients are not likely to take full care of their mouths during painful irradiation reactions; for irradiation produces a stomatitis, reduces further the blood supply of the periosteum and bone, decreases bone cell activity and resistance to infection. So with a poor dental condition already present the stage is set for pathogenic organisms to find their way between loosened teeth and the gum margins and thus proceed to the bone to set up an acute suppuration.

Because the extraction of teeth after heavy intraoral irradiation is an hazardous procedure it is more logical to remove all condemned teeth before such treatment. Otherwise they present a continuous peril to the patient cured of cancer; for during the ensuing years these teeth with their diminished blood supply will surely develop cavities, become soft, crumble or loosen, thus permitting introduction of infection into the devitalized maxilla in extractions. This may be the result as late as four years after treatment and cure of cancer.

Mechanical or chemical traumas such as the application of iodine to a healed intraoral irradiation scar have caused the onset of a fatal osteoradionecrosis of the mandible, so that three definite etiological factors are involved in the production of osteoradionecrosis: first, irradiation, then trauma followed by infection.

While all devitalized, loose and carious teeth should be removed before treatment, we must bear in mind that other teeth may later disintegrate due to the certain lack of adequate blood supply leading to eventual suppuration in the adjacent bone. This applies definitely to the teeth in the direct line of the applied radiation and thus the scientific discretion of the practitioner must determine the removal of such teeth as he may deem best for the welfare of the patient at the time and in the future. That is his responsibility, for the fullest knowledge of post-irradiation intraoral changes in the soft tissue and bone is highly essential when the subsequent problems of dentures, prosthetic appliances, dental hygiene and extractions arise.

---

[1] Watson, W. L., and Scarborough, J. E.: Osteoradionecrosis in Intra-oral Cancer, Am. Jour. Roentgenol. and Rad. Therapy, **40**, 524–534, 1938.

CHAPTER III.

INTRA-ORAL AND EXTRA-ORAL TECHNIQUE.

THE manufacturer of roentgen-ray equipment has ever striven to improve and perfect apparatus used to produce the roentgen-ray. From the discovery of this modern and beneficent phenomenon, down through the thirty odd years until the present day, they have labored to make and furnish the apparatus in form and construction to meet all possible requirements, and they have succeeded in presenting a product today which is highly standardized to an eminent degree of perfection. The roentgenologist and the manufacturer have contrived to reduce the size and to simplify equipment. The greatest stride in this direction did not come, however, until the World War, when Coolidge placed a radiator on the anode terminal on the outside of the tube and found the tube would rectify itself as long as the temperature of the tube was maintained below an uncertain degree. This discovery enabled the manufacturer to discard the bulky rectifying switches and the synchronous motor. Improvement in the design of the transformer, and the use of an auto-transformer instead of the rheostat, also helped in making our modern equipment so compact. Now we have equipment so portable that it may be carried into the home of the patient. This improvement may be attributed partly to the World War. Machines were often used as far forward as the field hospital. Naturally portability was an important factor in transportation, and this emergency was finally met by the discovery of the action of the Coolidge radiator tube.

Dr. W. D. Coolidge, the inventor of the Coolidge tube, discovered that if a very small Coolidge tube were immersed in oil along with the transformer, the oil would not only insulate the tube and transformer but would also radiate the tube. His patent application covering this principle bears the official dating of January 24, 1919. So that today we have two types of equipment for the dental office, each having its peculiar virtues. Of course, each has its peculiar faults as well, for no equipment is faultless. But today the dentist may obtain far better roentgen-ray apparatus than could have been obtained five years ago.

(66)

The following illustration of two of the most popular types of apparatus will give an idea of their construction. (Figs. 23 to 29.)

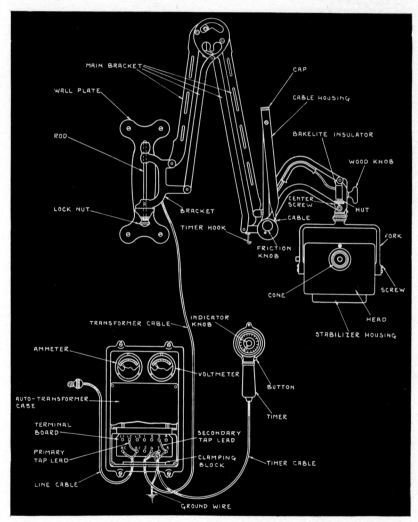

FIG. 23.—Victor C.D.X. dental roentgen-ray unit.

ROENTGENOLOGIC QUALIFICATIONS.

"A little learning is a dangerous thing." And particularly is this terse truism applicable to roentgenology, for in this special field of practice there can be no such distinction as a "slight degree" of error, for all errors, however slight, are grave. A faulty technique in the making of a roentgenogram, from the angulation of the tubes, of the apparatus and through the placement of the film packet, the

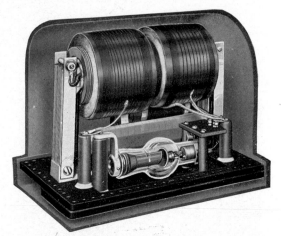

Fig. 24.—Phantom view of C.D.X. head.

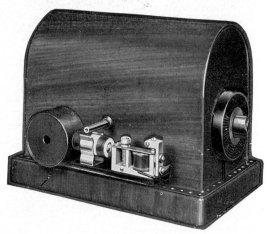

Fig. 25.—Showing Victor-Kearsley stabilizer.

development of the negative, the printing and the drying; or an error in interpretation of the finished product, howsoever clear-appearing, may cause untold suffering. The number of faulty roentgenograms that have served to induce inaccurate interpretations exceed, perhaps, the myriad of mistaken interpretations based upon accurate negatives; but both conditions contribute largely to the number of patients finally finding their way to the capable clinicians of our universities and to our foremost roentgenologists and oral surgeons.

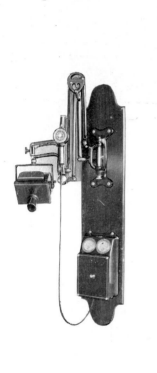

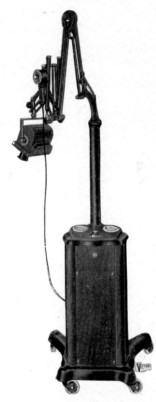

Fig. 26.—Victor C.D.X. dental roentgen-ray unit (wall type).

Fig. 27.—Victor C.D.X. dental roentgen-ray unit (mobile type).

It is not easy to interpret a perfect roentgenogram. It is impossible to interpret an imperfect one. The older system of mere clinical diagnosis having been superseded by the complementary addition of roentgenographic examination to assist and confirm it, neither method, alone, is sufficient today; and any roentgenogram of a standard less than perfect, or an interpretation less than thoroughly accurate, defeats its own purpose and renders valueless the most perfect clinical diagnosis.

Inexperience should preclude the ethical dentist from attempting the making or the interpretation of roentgenograms, and no one may claim to have achieved sufficient experience until he shall have

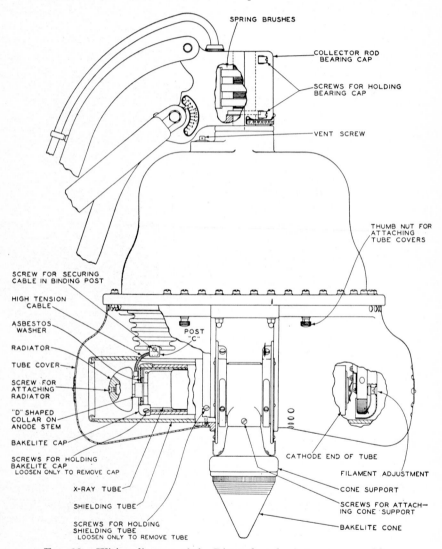

SPRING BRUSHES

COLLECTOR ROD BEARING CAP

SCREWS FOR HOLDING BEARING CAP

VENT SCREW

THUMB NUT FOR ATTACHING TUBE COVERS

SCREW FOR SECURING CABLE IN BINDING POST

HIGH TENSION CABLE

ASBESTOS WASHER

POST "C"

RADIATOR

TUBE COVER

SCREW FOR ATTACHING RADIATOR

"D" SHAPED COLLAR ON ANODE STEM

BAKELITE CAP

SCREWS FOR HOLDING BAKELITE CAP
LOOSEN ONLY TO REMOVE CAP

CATHODE END OF TUBE

FILAMENT ADJUSTMENT

X-RAY TUBE

CONE SUPPORT

SHIELDING TUBE

SCREWS FOR ATTACH-ING CONE SUPPORT

SCREWS FOR HOLDING SHIELDING TUBE
LOOSEN ONLY TO REMOVE TUBE

BAKELITE CONE

Fig. 28.—Wiring diagram of the Ritter dental roentgen-ray machine.

passed through an extensive period of training under the tutelage of patient, painstaking and capable instructors. This obvious

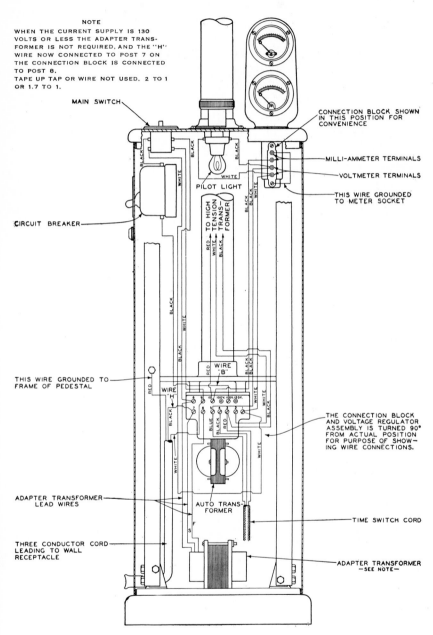

NOTE
WHEN THE CURRENT SUPPLY IS 130
VOLTS OR LESS THE ADAPTER TRANS-
FORMER IS NOT REQUIRED, AND THE "H"
WIRE NOW CONNECTED TO POST 7 ON
THE CONNECTION BLOCK IS CONNECTED
TO POST 8.
TAPE UP TAP OR WIRE NOT USED. 2 TO 1
OR 1.7 TO 1.

MAIN SWITCH

CONNECTION BLOCK SHOWN
IN THIS POSITION FOR
CONVENIENCE

MILLI-AMMETER TERMINALS

VOLTMETER TERMINALS

PILOT LIGHT

THIS WIRE GROUNDED
TO METER SOCKET

CIRCUIT BREAKER

RED — TO HIGH
WHITE TENSION
BLACK TRANS-
FORMER

WIRE "B"

THIS WIRE GROUNDED TO
FRAME OF PEDESTAL

WIRE "H"

THE CONNECTION BLOCK
AND VOLTAGE REGULATOR
ASSEMBLY IS TURNED 90°
FROM ACTUAL POSITION
FOR PURPOSE OF SHOW-
ING WIRE CONNECTIONS.

ADAPTER TRANSFORMER
LEAD WIRES

AUTO TRANS-
FORMER

TIME SWITCH CORD

THREE CONDUCTOR CORD
LEADING TO WALL
RECEPTACLE

ADAPTER TRANSFORMER
—SEE NOTE—

Fig. 29.—Head of machine containing transformer and X-ray tube, Ritter
dental roentgen-ray machine.

truth, unfortunately, has not deterred many unqualified dentists from persuading themselves that the main qualification of a roentgenologist is the possession of necessary equipment, a few instruc-

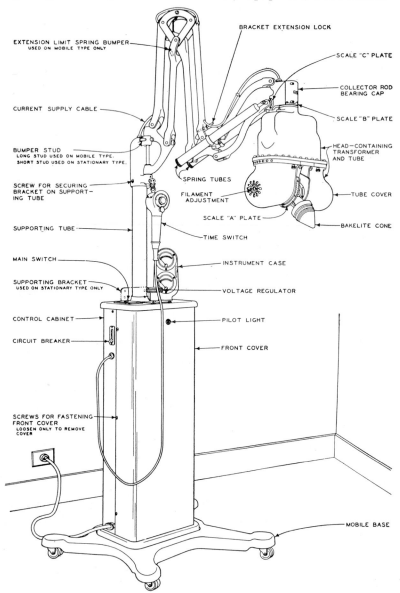

EXTENSION LIMIT SPRING BUMPER
USED ON MOBILE TYPE ONLY

BRACKET EXTENSION LOCK

SCALE "C" PLATE

COLLECTOR ROD
BEARING CAP

CURRENT SUPPLY CABLE

SCALE "B" PLATE

HEAD—CONTAINING
TRANSFORMER
AND TUBE

BUMPER STUD
LONG STUD USED ON MOBILE TYPE.
SHORT STUD USED ON STATIONARY TYPE.

SPRING TUBES

SCREW FOR SECURING
BRACKET ON SUPPORT—
ING TUBE

FILAMENT
ADJUSTMENT

TUBE COVER

SCALE "A" PLATE

SUPPORTING TUBE

BAKELITE CONE

TIME SWITCH

MAIN SWITCH

INSTRUMENT CASE

SUPPORTING BRACKET
USED ON STATIONARY TYPE ONLY

VOLTAGE REGULATOR

CONTROL CABINET

PILOT LIGHT

CIRCUIT BREAKER

FRONT COVER

SCREWS FOR FASTENING
FRONT COVER
LOOSEN ONLY TO REMOVE
COVER

MOBILE BASE

FIG. 30.—Ritter dental roentgen-ray machine.

tions on the method of using it, a descriptive explanation of the apparatus, and a general treatise on interpretation. And to this, probably, may be added a fearsome unwillingness to refer patients to a more eminent practitioner in the specialized field.

There can be no halfway methods. A roentgenogram cannot be partly wrong or partly inaccurate. The slightest inaccuracy nullifies its possible assistance in diagnosis, and this applies to whether it has been poorly made or even poorly developed, for an interpretation of such negatives is not merely impossible but they are always the source of danger in the hands of those who cannot recognize their defects immediately. Unfortunately there are many who cannot, but who still essay interpretations. There is no guessing about what a negative shows, for the value of the roentgenogram is entirely gone where guesses and doubts interpose. The interpretation of roentgenograms should never be attempted without the firmest foundation of knowledge of the histological, anatomical, and pathological conditions present in any area under observation. The most delicate part of the tissues and structures must be intimately and thoroughly understood; for otherwise there would be no ability to differentiate between the normal and abnormal conditions possibly appearing, and sometimes the fine hair-line differences are almost microscopic, but must be recognized. The mere suggestion of this necessary qualification should indicate the more than superficial knowledge demanded of the operator, and should impress again that the mere installation of equipment in an office no more qualifies a dentist as a roentgenologist than the possession of authoritative books on painting would qualify one as an artist.

To that phase of roentgenology covering a field of examinations wherein the film is placed inside of the mouth, and whereby usually is attained a detail of conditions surrounding the individual teeth, we apply the term "intra-oral roentgenography." It is merely a term of classification to distinguish the cases so examined from those requiring that the film be on the outside of the mouth, as is necessary where a greater area must be examined. Fracture of the jaw, tumors, cysts, osteomyelitis, foreign bodies and other grosser conditions represent the type of cases requiring a technique which we term "extra-oral roentgenography."

One of the most worrisome moments in the life of the roentgenologist is when he is asked to interpret a roentgenogram made by another; for however clean and clear the negative, the exact conditions under which it was made cannot be assumed by the interpreter to have been perfect without having the most intimate knowledge of the ability and experience of the operator. Any negative that indicates a deviation from the absolute, the accurate, the natural figure or area represented is a distortion. An interpreter with a deeply comprehensive knowledge of anatomical structures may detect distortions that quickly indicate to the trained eye and mind an unusual bulk, or size, or position of an object, and yet every line on the negative might appear to confirm a clinical diagnosis of a pathological condition that had no existence. A shadow appearing in the apical region, or one surrounding a root canal, may be considered with justifiable significance in many cases merely from the registrations on the negative; but we must first be convinced that these shadows are not distortions due to errors in angulation at which the rays were directed. That does happen more than seldom; and there are many other ways for distortions to creep into a roentgenogram. Almost any attempt to compromise with precise technique may cause a distortion to trouble the interpreter. Uncertain manipulation, unscientific handling of the delicate mechanism of a roentgen-ray apparatus in sending those intense rays through the delicate structures and tissues of the oral cavity may show on the film suggestions of conditions that really have no existence. They may appear in the negative as clear indications of a pathological involvement, whereas they are distortions that take a thorough student of anatomical, histological, and pathological conditions to discern with certainty; and the greatest trouble, the real pernicious aspect, is that the slightest distortions work the heaviest distress because of the difficulty of their detection.

So the roentgenologist, from among all the principles of technique that have been framed to guide him, should select as the cardinal aim of his efforts the avoidance of distortion on roentgenograms; for if distortion be not avoided his efforts will be not only valueless, but, as probably, harmful.

To prevent distortion, the first step is the proper placement of the roentgen-ray tube in relation to the point under examination and to the film. Perfected roentgenographic equipment permits the movement of the tube in only two planes, allowing the angles at which the tube may be set within either plane to be figured quickly and accurately and to be adjusted easily. The two planes are distinct opposites: a vertical plane and a horizontal plane.

The horizontal plane in which the tube moves is always certain: it is parallel with the level of the floor. So, to attain a true technique, there must be found a plane of the head that also is parallel with the plane of the floor. That, naturally, we find in the plane of occlusion; but before any of the rules governing the angulation of the tube may be followed, it is necessary that the head of the subject be in a position so that the plane of occlusion is absolutely parallel with the plane of the floor.

In this horizontal plane, which we have defined, the tube so moves that all of its motion is around a perpendicular from the plane of the floor; and, consequently, if we are to make use of it, there must be established a plane of the head that is perpendicular to the plane of the floor. The sagittal plane answers that requirement, designating the vertical plane in which the tube moves. And thus, in the vertical plane, however we adjust the tube, it will always move in a manner to form an angle, sometimes plus and sometimes minus, with the plane of occlusion.

So, to secure the necessary position for the penetration of rays issuing through the tube, the patient should be placed so that, sitting in a chair, not only is the plane of occlusion parallel to the plane of the floor, but that the sagittal plane forms a true parallel to a perpendicular from the plane of the floor.

Having the limiting planes within which the tube moves, the horizontal and the vertical as represented by the occlusal and the sagittal planes of the head, the angulation of the tube looms as the important function because the slightest deviation from the proper direction can cause so much distress from distortions appearing on the negative. There are fine shades in distinctions of angulation in special cases that no set rule could possibly govern the experienced roentgenologist; there are cases where as many as six or eight exposures may be made at the identical same point before the best results are obtained under rays directed at one particular angle. But there are governing rules of angulation that control absolutely the fundamental technique of roentgenology, and without a strict obedience to these rules in the roentgenologic examination of teeth, the operator will fail.

RULES GOVERNING ANGULATION.

1. The tube must be so set that the direct rays are perpendicular to the mean tangent of the teeth under examination.

2. Bisect the angle formed by the mean plane of the film and the mean plane of the tooth, and direct the rays perpendicular to the bisecting plane. (Fig. 31.)

The first rule enunciated must be followed if anterior-posterior distortions are to be escaped; for unless the direct rays pass perfectly perpendicular to the mean tangent of the teeth, the negative

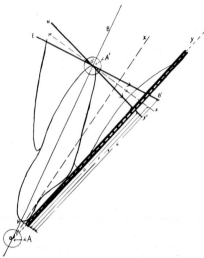

FIG. 31.—Cieszynski's "rule of isometry." Line *O–B*, mean plane of tooth; line *O–Y*, plane of film; line *O–X*, bisecting < *A;* line *E–B'*, rays perpendicular to line *O–B;* distance *G*, greater than *H–O'* (elongation); line *N–Y'*, rays perpendicular to line *O–Y;* distance *D*, less than *H–O*, (foreshortening); line *M–X'*, rays perpendicular to line *O–X;* distance *F'* equals line *H–O* (correct).

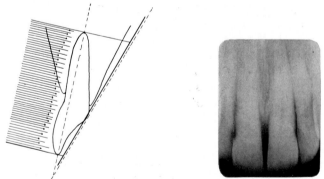

FIG. 32.—Rays directed perpendicular to the plane of the tooth resulting in longitudinal or distortion of the root.

will not give the true anterior-posterior dimensions. And likewise, neither may the second rule, called the "rule of isometry" by

Cieszynski, who first formulated it (1907), be disregarded in the smallest degree. For if, instead of directing our rays perpendicular to the bisecting plane, we direct the rays perpendicular to the mean plane of the tooth, we would surely derive an elongation, a longitudinal distortion, to render an interpretation and a diagnosis impossible. (Fig. 32.)

INTRA-ORAL ROENTGENOLOGY.

If the rays are directed perpendicularly to the mean plane of the film (Fig. 33), we get a foreshortening. But by following faithfully the basic rule enunciated, directing the rays halfway

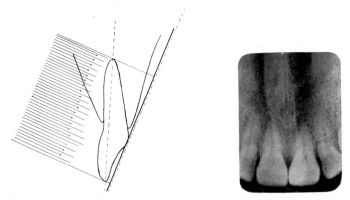

FIG. 33.—Rays directed perpendicular to the plane of the film resulting in foreshortening of the root.

between these two planes so as to be perpendicular to the bisecting plane (Figs. 34 and 35), we obtain a result as nearly perfect as possible under the present state of the science.

The essential factors are the sagittal plane of the head, the occlusal plane of the teeth, the horizontal plane in which the tube moves, and the vertical plane in which the tube moves. These planes are most important, and they bear a definite working relationship to each other: The tube moving in a horizontal plane around the sagittal plane of the head, and the tube moving in a vertical plane from the occlusal plane of the teeth, are the major movements that are so highly important in the prevention of longitudinal and vertical distortion.

The sagittal plane of the head must be perpendicular to the plane of the floor at all times. (Fig. 36.) It matters not whether the head is tilted forward, or tilted backward in such a position that the occlusal plane is perpendicular to the floor, the sagittal plane

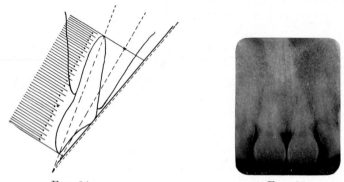

Fig. 34   Fig. 35

FIGS. 34 and 35.—Rays directed perpendicular to the bisecting plane resulting in the correct shadow of the teeth.

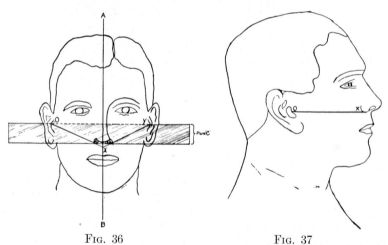

Fig. 36   Fig. 37

FIG. 36.—*A–B*, the sagittal plane, must always be perpendicular to the floor. Plane *C*, the occlusal plane, must always be parallel to the floor.

FIG. 37.—*O–X* is the line of orientation for the maxillary teeth.

must remain perpendicular. It is the first step in the production of a roentgenogram and a most important one, as any deviation of this plane to the right or left seriously affects the angulation.

The occlusal plane of the teeth must be *parallel* with the plane of the floor at all times. (Fig. 36.) If we take an imaginary line from the tragus of the ear to the ala of the nose and establish that line parallel with the floor, we will find that the plane of occlusion of the maxillary teeth is parallel to the floor (Fig. 37), for they are parallel to each other. But when the mouth is opened the occlusal plane of the lower teeth changes its position and, therefore, is not parallel to the floor. So to place the occlusal plane of the mandibular teeth in proper relationship to the floor it is necessary to tilt the head backward. (Fig. 38.) The occlusal plane of the mandibu-

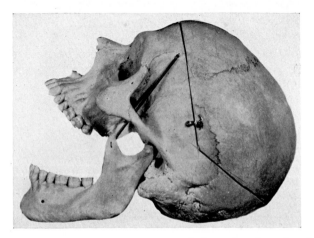

Fig. 38.—Head tilted back, mouth opened, in order that the plane of occlusion of the mandibular teeth may be parallel to the floor.

lar teeth will then be brought forward and upward until the plane of occlusion becomes parallel with the floor. This may be judged by eye. However, if one wished to be absolutely sure these planes are in their proper positions, they may do so by placing an occlusal plane leveler (Fig. 39) in the mouth, the proper position of the planes being indicated by the spirit level.

It may readily be seen, therefore, that if the sagittal plane and the occlusal plane are perpendicular and parallel to the floor respectively, the head is divided into four quarters (Fig. 40), and that a definite position of the head has been established. So now may be considered the movement of the tube in its relationship to these planes.

The roentgen-ray tube moving in two planes, the horizontal and the vertical, their definite relationship to the planes of the head must ever be in mind.

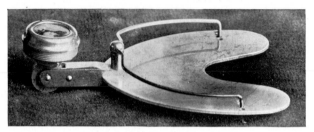

FIG. 39.—Occlusal plane leveler.

The tube moves in a horizontal plane around the sagittal plane (Fig. 41), and the proper relationship between these planes must be maintained at all times so as to prevent a mesial or distal dis-

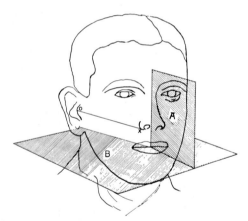

FIG. 40.—Head divided into four quarters by the sagittal plane (A) and the occlusal plane (B).

tortion. (Fig. 42.) In order to give a complete diagnosis without resorting to guesswork it is necessary to make at least fourteen exposures (Fig. 43), seven for the maxillary teeth and seven for the mandibular teeth, and the horizontal position of the tube must be perpendicular to the mean tangent of the teeth involved. (Fig. 44.)

The horizontal position of the tube for the various teeth is as follows: Having the direct rays parallel with the floor, they are directed perpendicularly to the sagittal plane for the molar region (Figs. 48 and 61.) As the teeth form a curved arch, all teeth will

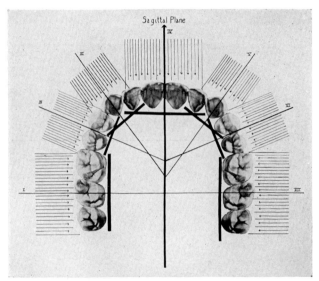

FIG. 41.—Direction of rays perpendicular to the mean tangents of the teeth to be examined.

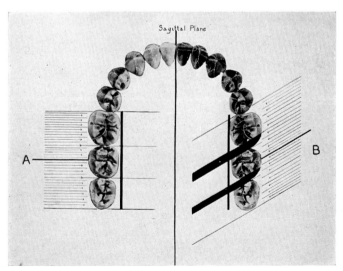

FIG. 42.—*A*, proper relationship between rays and the mean tangent of the teeth. *B*, incorrect relationship between the rays and the teeth.

6

not have the same tangent. It may easily be seen that the mean tangents of the premolar teeth are not the same as that of the molars, and the tangents of the canine and incisors are not the same as that of the premolars. Naturally the horizontal movement of the

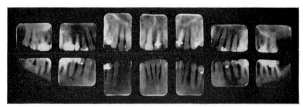

Fig. 43.—Showing a complete roentgenographic examination of the mouth (fourteen films). Illustrating the relative position of the film to the long axis of the teeth.

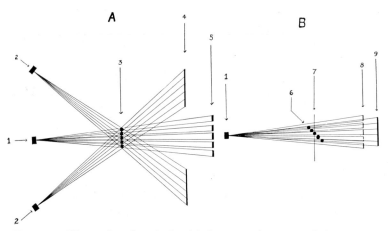

Fig. 44.—Illustrating the relationship between the rays and the tangents of the teeth. *A:* 1, source of the rays; 3, mean tangents of five balls representing the mean tangents of the teeth (in this relationship the resultant shadows of the balls are separate and distinct); 5, if the source of light is changed to position 2, the shadows of the balls merge, with the result that only one shadow is produced, 4. *B:* 1, source of rays constant with the mean tangent of the balls changed from 7 to 6. Result shows that instead of having individual shadows, 8, we have only one shadow, 9.

tube must be adjusted so as to be perpendicular to these various tangents, and the tube must be moved anteriorly at an angle of 10 degrees from the perpendicular (as used in the molar region) for the premolars. (Figs. 53 and 64.) And for the canine region, the tube is moved in the horizontal plane until it is at an angle of 45 degrees to a perpendicular from the sagittal plane. (Figs. 56 and 66.) Further, as we come to the first and second incisors, the tube is placed to allow the rays to parallel the sagittal plane. (Figs. 58 and 68.)

The movement of the tube in the horizontal plane is the same for both the maxilla (Fig. 47) and the mandible (Fig. 60), as the curve of the mandibular teeth generally follows that of the teeth of the maxilla. This is true in all cases except where abnormal conditions appear.

From the plane of occlusion the tube moves in a perpendicular plane, starting at 0 degrees. Cieszynski's rule of isometry governs the extent of movement of the tube in the vertical plane.

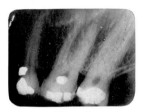
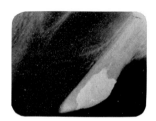

| Fig. 45 | Fig. 46 |

Figs. 45 and 46.—Illustrating anterior-posterior distortion, the result of incorrect relationship between the teeth and the rays in the horizontal plane.

Assuming the tube properly adjusted in the horizontal plane, the adjustment of the tube in the vertical plane is as follows: If lines drawn parallel with the long axis of the teeth were continued beyond the apical region, they would meet at a common point. In the normal maxilla the axes of the anterior teeth have a slight distal inclination, while the premolars and molars are inclined toward the sagittal plane. This inclination, combined with the fact that the palatine vault is much higher in the posterior portion than in the anterior, naturally governs the position of the film in its relationship to the mean plane of the teeth. One can readily realize that the vertical position of the tube cannot be the same for the molars as it would be for the anterior teeth. In the molar region, therefore, as the plane of the film and the plane of the teeth are near parallel, the tube is raised in a vertical plane to any angu-

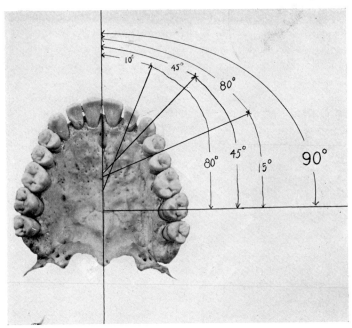

FIG. 47.—Horizontal movement of the tube demonstrating the various angles in the plane of occlusion.

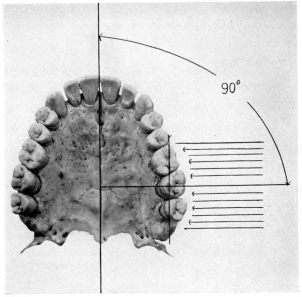

FIG. 48.—Angulation of the horizontal movement of the tube for the molar region of the maxilla.

lation of from 25 to 30 degrees. (Fig. 49.) In the premolar region the wall of the vault curving around the sagittal plane, and the plane of the teeth converging toward the sagittal plane to a greater degree than in the molar region, the vertical angle of the tube becomes greater and the tube must be set at 35 degrees. (Fig. 54.) These conditions become more acute as we arrive at the canine

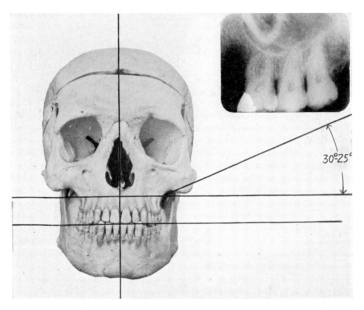

Fig. 49.—Angulation of the vertical movement of the tube for the molar region of the maxilla.

region, where the vertical angle of the tube is placed at 45 to 50 degrees. (Fig. 57.) And as we find the conditions which govern the relationship of the film and teeth most acute in the anterior portion of the mouth, the vertical angle varies between 55 and 65 degrees (Fig. 59), all angles being measured from the occlusal plane.

In the mandible the planes of all teeth are practically the same, that is, perpendicular to the plane of occlusion. Here, however, it is a change in the depth of the floor of the mouth which regulates the vertical angle of the tube. In the molar region of the mandible the floor of the mouth being very deep, it enables placing the film in the mouth in such a position that the plane of the film and the plane of the teeth are parallel. Therefore, the vertical angle of the tube

for the lower molars is 0 degrees. (Fig. 62.) In the premolar region
the floor of the mouth being shallower, when the film is placed in this
region the lower portion of the film naturally slopes toward the

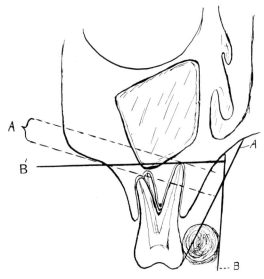

Fig. 50.—Le Masters' technique for the elimination of the malar process
in roentgenograms of the molar region. *A*, film in normal position; *B*, film
with cotton roll attached, the rays, *B'*, directed below the process.

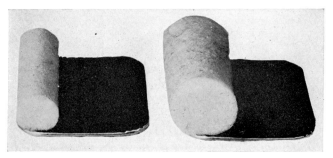

Fig. 51.—Film with cotton roll attached, ready for use.

sagittal plane; and, applying the rule of isometry, we find it necessary to drop our tube in the vertical plane to a −10 degrees. (Fig.
65.) As we near the sagittal plane, the floor of the mouth in the
anterior portion being very shallow, the bisecting angle is greater

in this region than in the premolar region. So it becomes necessary to change the vertical angle of the tube for the mandibular canine and incisors to a −20 degrees. (Figs. 67 and 69.) All these angles are measured from the occlusal plane.

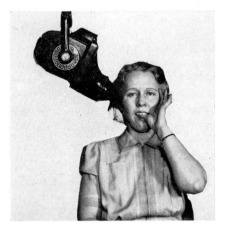

FIG. 52.—Film being held in place with the thumb. The fingers placed on the side of the face prevent movement of the film and steady the hand.

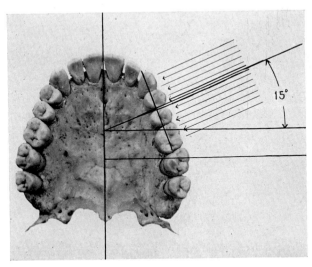

FIG. 53.—Angulation of the horizontal movement of the tube for the premolar region of the maxilla.

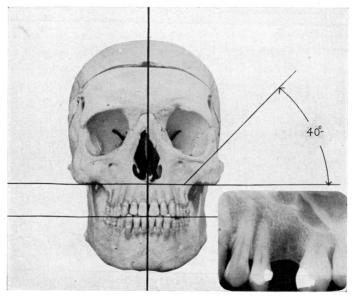

FIG. 54.—Angulation of the vertical movement of the tube for the premolar region of the maxilla.

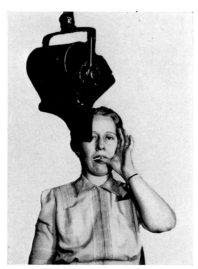

FIG. 55.—Film being held in place with the thumb. The fingers on the side of the face prevent the movement of the film.

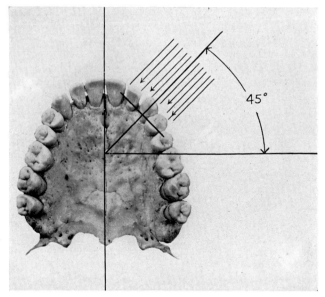

Fig. 56.—Angulation of the horizontal movement of the tube for the canine region of the maxilla.

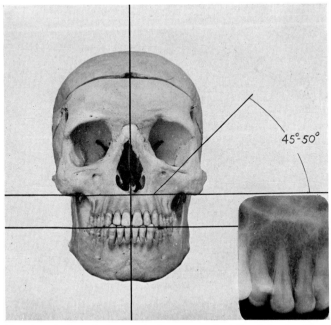

Fig. 57.—Angulation of the vertical movement of the tube for the canine region of the maxilla.

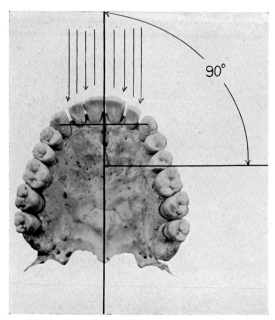

Fig. 58.—Angulation of the horizontal movement of the tube for the region of the incisors of the maxilla.

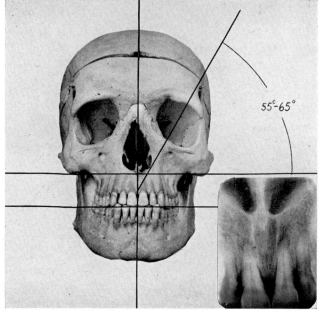

Fig. 59.—Angulation of the vertical movement of the tube for the region of the incisors of the maxilla.

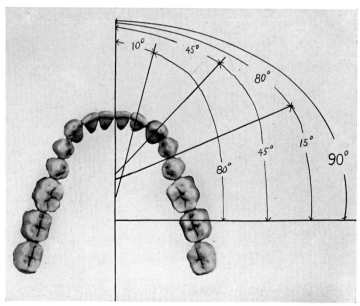

Fig. 60.—Horizontal movement of the tube demonstrating the various angles for the mandible in the plane of occlusion.

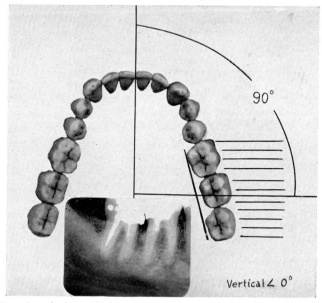

Fig. 61.—Angulation of the horizontal movement of the tube for the molar region of the mandible.

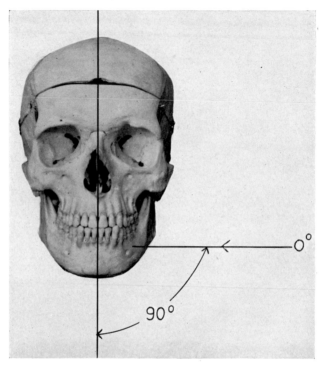

FIG. 62.—Angulation of the vertical movement of the tube for the molar region of the mandible.

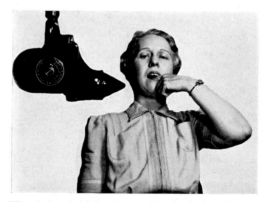

FIG. 63.—Film being held in place with the index finger. The side of the hand resting against the face, and a lateral pressure being exerted against the film. The arm is thrown completely out of the way and does not interfere with the operator and in this position allows a more direct force to be applied to the film.

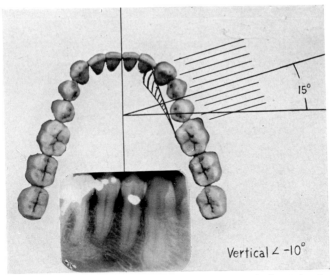

Fig. 64.—Angulation of the horizontal movement of the tube for the premolar region of the mandible.

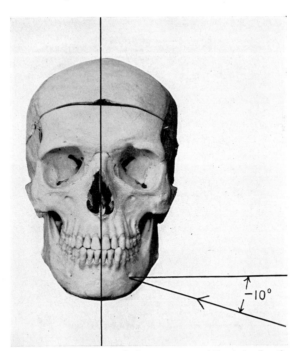

Fig. 65.—Angulation of the vertical movement of the tube for the premolar region of the mandible.

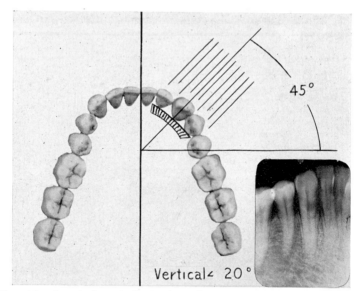

Fig. 66.—Angulation of the horizontal movement of the tube for the canine region of the mandible.

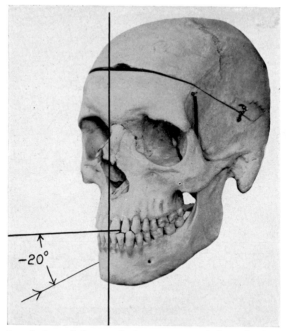

Fig. 67.—Angulation of the vertical movement of the tube for the canine region of the mandible.

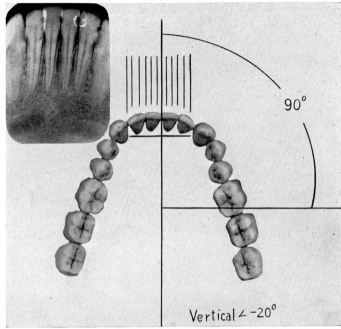

Fig. 68.—Angulation of the horizontal movement of the tube for the region of the incisors of the mandible.

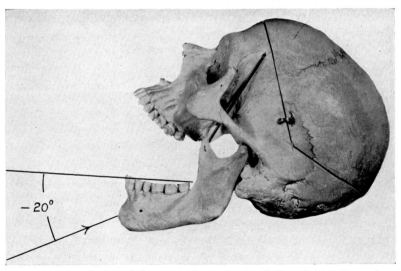

Fig. 69.—Angulation of the vertical movement of the tube for the region of the incisors of the mandible.

Having the sagittal plane perpendicular to the floor, and the plane of occlusion parallel to the floor, the angles of the tube for the various parts of the mouth are as follows:

	Horizontal plane, degrees.	Vertical plane, degrees.
Maxilla:		
Molar region	0	25 to 30
Premolar region	15	35
Canine region	45	45
Incisor region	90	55 to 65
Mandible:		
Molar region	0	0
Premolar region	15	−10
Canine region	45	−20
Incisor region	90	−20

Once the head is placed in the proper position and the tube is adjusted to the correct angulation, there remains but two operations to be carried out: (1) The placement of the tube so that the central rays are directed at the apex of the teeth, and (2) the duration of exposure.

If we draw a line from the tragus of the ear to the ala of the nose and cut through on this plane, we would pass through the apical region of the maxillary teeth (Fig. 76); so in making exposures of the maxillary teeth, the central rays should pass through, or be over, this line. The point of entry of our direct rays for the mandibular teeth is 0.5 cm. above the lower border of the mandible.

To localize the penetration-point for the teeth of the maxilla, the planes being in their proper positions, a line is dropped from the outer canthus of the eye so that it crosses the plane of occlusion at right angles. This line passes through the first molar; and where this line crosses the imaginary line drawn from the tragus of the ear to the ala of the nose (Fig. 76) will be found the apical region of the first molar; and the central rays must be directed at that intersection. The apical region of the second molar is 1 cm. distal, and that of the third molar 2 cm. distal from the region of the first molar.

The premolars are localized by bisecting the eye and dropping a line perpendicular to the plane of occlusion; and it crosses our imaginary line, which is parallel with the plane of occlusion, between the apices of the first and second premolars. Therefore, for the premolars, the rays must be centered over this intersection. The apex of the canine will be on this same line 5 mm. distal to the ala of the nose, while the incisor will be found by directing the rays through the nasal fossa. (Fig. 77.)

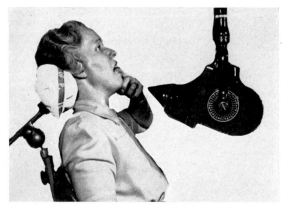

FIG. 70.—Correct position of the hand, film, head and tube for roentgenograms of the lower incisors.

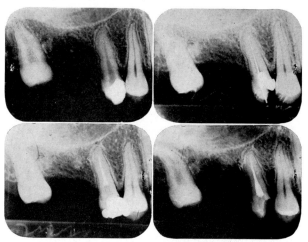

FIG. 71.—Reproduction of an area by following the foregoing technique.

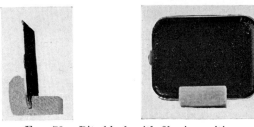

FIG. 72.—Bite-block with film in position.

7

Localizing the teeth of the mandible is less intricate because it is easier to see into the mouth and direct the rays accordingly. However, the same landmarks as used for localizing the teeth in the maxilla may be used in the mandible.

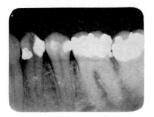
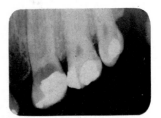

Fig. 73   Fig. 74

Fig. 73.—Roentgenogram produced in conjunction with the bite-block demonstrating the amount of film above the occlusal surfaces of the teeth which is wasted. This wasted film could be used to great advantage in the apical region of the teeth as the area beyond the apex is not shown.

Fig. 74.—Roentgenogram of the molar region, showing the distal portion of the film out of line. This condition is caused by improper placement of the film and failure to hold the film correctly.

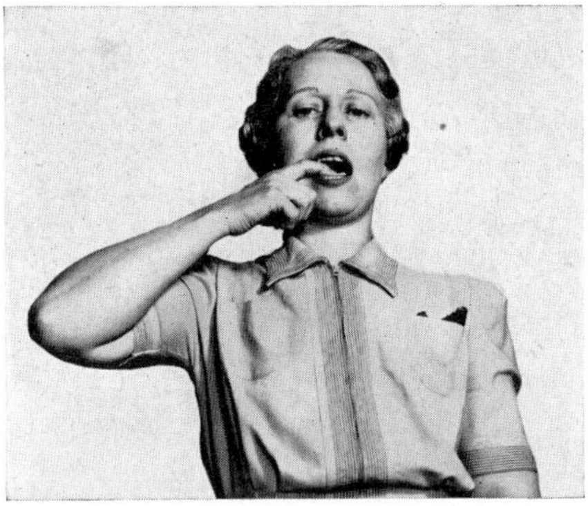

Fig. 75.—Film held in the proper position. The upper border of the film should be on a level with the incisal margins of the teeth.

Very often, due to the prominences of the malar bone, rays projected in the maxillary molar region at the normal angulation will superimpose a dense shadow of the malar bone upon the roots of the molars. Sometimes the shadow is so dense as to prevent the appearance of the apical regions of the molars upon the film.

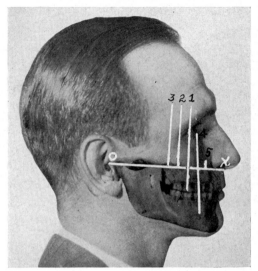

Fig. 76.—*O—X* is the line of orientation. 1, where lines cross is point of entry for the first molar; 2, point of entry for the second molar; 3, point of entry for the third molar; 4, point of entry for the premolars; 5, point of entry for the canine.

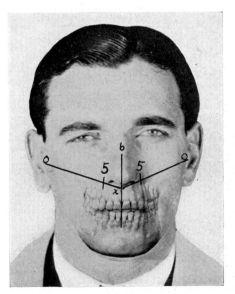

Fig. 77.—5, point of entry for the canine; 6, point of entry for the incisors.

This condition may be overcome by following the technique originated by LeMasters, who fastened a cotton roll (Fig. 51) to the emulsion side of the film packet, so that when the packet is inserted into the oral cavity the cotton roll rests against the lingual surface of the molars, held in position by the thumb of the patient. The thumb of the hand on the side opposite from which the operator is working will be used.

This permits the mean plane of the film to lie more perpendicularly to the mean plane of the teeth than would be the case if the film rested directly against the lingual surface of the teeth; and so we may decrease the angulation of the rays sufficiently to avoid their penetration of the malar bone (Fig. 50), thus eliminating the shadow of the malar bone in the roentgenogram.

TECHNIQUE OF THE OCCLUSAL FILM.

There are often pathological conditions in the mouth of so gross a nature that the small intra-oral films are insufficient in size to outline the lesion. This makes necessary a resort to a film accommodating the need. A film suitable for the purpose, and at the same time available for smaller intra-oral demands, is known as the Bite Film (Eastman occlusal film). With it may be located impacted teeth, supernumerary teeth, cysts, odontomes, fractures of the mandible, and also stones in Wharton's duct which may exist in the floor of the mouth.

Maxilla.—The film is inserted in the mouth, the emulsion facing the palate, between the occlusal surfaces of the teeth in the plane of occlusion. The film should be eased back in the mouth until the posterior border of the film packet is in contact with the tissues over the anterior border of the ramus. Adjust the head of the patient so as to have the sagittal plane perpendicular to the floor and the occlusal plane parallel to the floor. This naturally will bring the plane of the film parallel to the floor.

For an examination of the anterior region of the palate the tube is moved in the horizontal plane until the central rays are parallel with the sagittal plane, and moved in the vertical plane until the central rays are 65 degrees to the plane of occlusion. (Fig. 78.) For the small dental units, the time of exposure is usually seven seconds, giving the result as seen in Figs. 79 and 80.

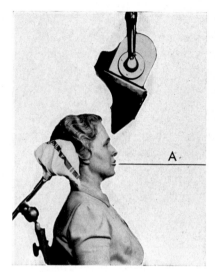

FIG. 78.—Relationship of the tube to the plane of the film for roentgeno-grams of the palate, using the Eastman occlusal film. (*A*) the plane of occlusion maintained at a parallel with the floor plane.

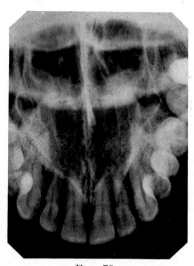

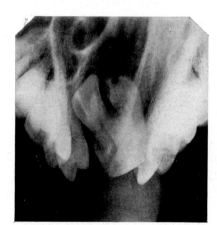

FIG. 79   FIG. 80

FIGS. 79 and 80.—Two roentgenograms, taken according to the technique as shown in Fig. 78.

For the canine region the horizontal angle of the tube should be set at 45 degrees to the sagittal plane, and the vertical angle 65 degrees to the plane of occlusion (Fig. 81), the central rays directed

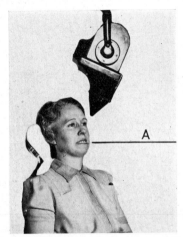

Fig. 81.—Relationship of the tube to the plane of the film for roentgenograms of the canine region of the palate, using Eastman occlusal film. Direct rays passing through the canine fossa. (*A*) the plane of occlusion maintained at a parallel with the floor.

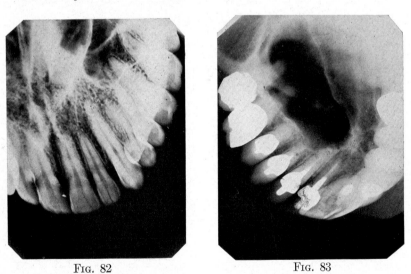

Fig. 82   Fig. 83

Figs. 82 and 83.—Roentgenograms taken according to the technique as shown in Fig. 81.

through the canine region, giving the results as seen in Figs. 82 and 83. The time of exposure should be the same as for the anterior region, seven seconds.

It is often necessary to obtain a roentgenogram of this type in the maxillary molar region. In such cases the horizontal angle of the tube should be set at 90 degrees to the sagittal plane and the

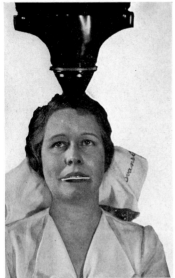 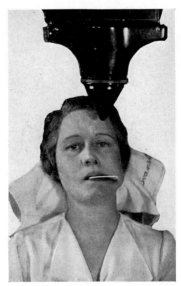

| FIG. 84 | FIG. 85 |

FIG. 84.—The patient's head placed so that the plane of occlusion is parallel to the plane of the floor; the film placed in the mouth posteriorly as far as permitted by the patient; the direct rays are positioned to parallel the sagittal plane.

FIG. 85.—The head maintained in position, the plane of occlusion parallel with the floor, the film is shifted laterally until the inner border of the film is parallel with the sagittal plane; the tube is shifted so that the direct rays parallel the sagittal plane but pass through the infra-orbital foramen.

vertical angle of the tube at from 60 to 70 degrees. The exposure-time must then be advanced to eight seconds, which will give the result seen in Figs. 607 and 608.

For intra-oral examination of the maxillary sinuses to supplement the extra-oral technique suggested herein we should resort to the occlusal film.

The patient is placed in the chair in position to bring the sagittal plane of the head perpendicular to the floor, and the plane of occlusion parallel with the floor.

Film is then placed in the mouth as far posteriorly as possible, its emulsion side toward the palate (Fig. 84), then carried laterally until the inner border of the film packet is on a line with the sagittal plane. (Fig. 85.)

In this position we find the maxillary sinus directly over the film, and the tube is placed in position so that the direct rays parallel the sagittal plane (Fig. 84) and is then shifted laterally until the central rays will pass through the infra-orbital foramen. (Fig. 85.)

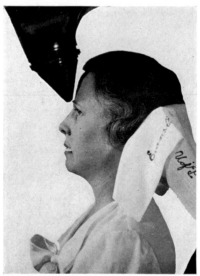

Fig. 86.—The plane of occlusion is parallel with the floor, the film in proper position. The vertical angulation of the tube is adjusted to read between 75 degrees and 85 degrees, depending upon the distal slope of the patients forehead.

The vertical angulation of the tube should be somewhere between 75 and 85 degrees, depending upon the slope of the forehead, with the direct rays passing through the infra-orbital foramen. (Fig. 86.) For patients having decidedly receding foreheads, the vertical angle of the tube may be set at approximately 85 degrees.

This type of examination will aid in differentiating cystic areas from the maxillary sinus, and will also reveal any residual roots in the sinus. (Figs. 87, 88, 89, 90 and 91.)

Mandible.—The film is prepared and placed in the mouth in the manner similar to that followed in the maxilla, except that the emulsion side of the film would in these cases face the floor of the mouth.

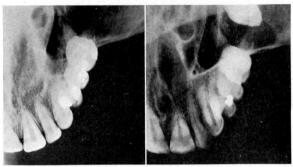

Fig. 87   Fig. 88

Figs. 87 and 88.—Roentgenograms showing the floor of the maxillary sinus made by following the technique described in Figs. 84, 85, and 86.

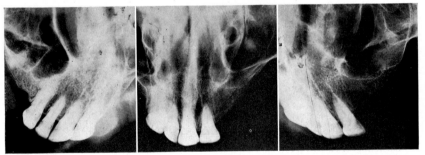

Fig. 89   Fig. 90   Fig. 91

Figs. 89, 90 and 91.—Three roentgenograms of the same patient revealing residual roots in the walls of both the right and left maxillary sinuses. Figs. 89 and 90 were taken at an angle of 65 degrees through the canine fossa as described in Fig. 81; while Fig. 90 was taken with the direct rays paralleling the sagittal plane as described in Figs. 84, 85 and 86, which gives more accurate information of the position of the roots.

For an examination of the mandible in the region of the symphysis, the sagittal plane of the head is placed perpendicular to the floor; the chair is now tilted backward until the plane of occlusion is 45 degrees to the plane of the floor. Thereupon the tube is manipulated in the horizontal plane until the central rays are parallel to the

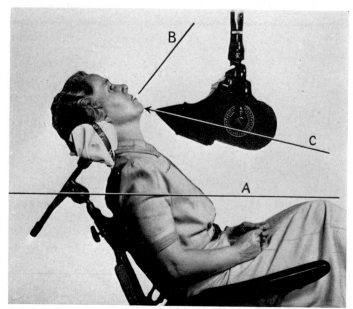

Fig. 92.—Relationship of the tube to the plane of the film for roentgenograms of the region embracing the symphysis of the mandible, using Eastman occlusal film. Direct rays are parallel to the sagittal plane. (*B*) Plane of occlusion forty-five (45) degrees to the plane of the floor; (*A*) line parallel with the plane of the floor; (*C*) vertical angulation of the tube minus fifteen (—15) degrees

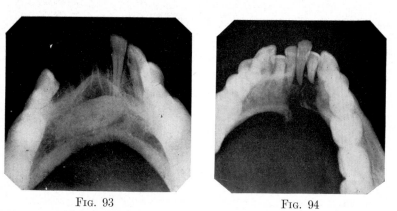

Fig. 93   Fig. 94

Figs. 93 and 94.—Roentgenograms taken according to the technique as shown in Fig. 92, revealing an impacted canine (Fig. 93) and a fracture of the symphysis (Fig. 94).

sagittal plane, and adjusted in the vertical plane until the central rays are at −15 degrees to the plane of the floor. From this position the central rays are directed through the symphysis (Fig. 92) for an exposure-time of seven seconds, giving a result as seen in Figs. 93 and 94.

It often becomes necessary to examine minutely the floor of the mouth. Especially is this imperative when attempting to localize stones in Wharton's duct.

To examine this region the chair must be tilted backward until

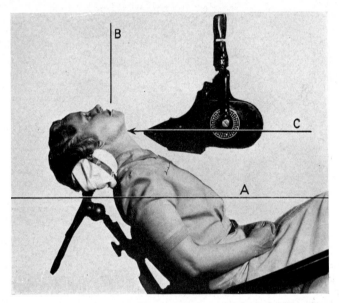

Fig. 95.—Relationship of the tube to the plane of the film for roentgenograms of the floor of the mouth, using Eastman occlusal film. (*C*) Direct rays perpendicular to the plane of the film and parallel to the sagittal plane; (*B*) plane of occlusion perpendicular to the floor; (*A*) plane of the floor.

the occlusal plane is perpendicular to the plane of the floor (Fig. 95); and thereupon the tube manipulated in the horizontal plane until the rays are parallel to the sagittal plane, and manipulated in the vertical plane until the rays are perpendicular to the occlusal plane. (Fig. 95.) On account of the rays being called to penetrate no osseous structure, save only the pathological lesion, the time of exposure may be reduced to six seconds, and the result will be as indicated in Fig. 96.

This is the only satisfactory practical method known for such cases, for by it is avoided any superimposing, a result so often encountered when using lateral plates where the stone was thereby prevented from showing in so many instances.

RAPER BITE-WING FILM.

The bite-wing film packet bears a small tab attached to and extending from the center of its emulsion side; and when in the

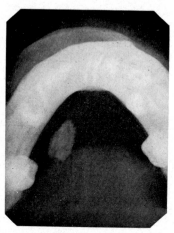

FIG. 96.—Roentgenogram taken according to the technique shown in Fig. 95, revealing a stone in Wharton's duct.

mouth, this tab, resting between the occlusal surfaces of the teeth, holds the film in contact with the lingual surfaces of the teeth under examination.

The head of the patient must lie in the head-rest of the chair so that the plane of occlusion will be parallel to the floor, the sagittal plane being perpendicular to the floor. Place the tube at 10 degrees in the vertical plane, at which angulation it should be for all exposures with the bite-wing films. The horizontal movement of the tube is the guiding factor, and the basic general rules for preventing an anterior-posterior distortion must be strictly followed. So the horizontal angulation of the tube should be the same as used in other intra-oral examinations, and, therefore, will be moved in the horizontal plane so that it rests in a position perpendicular to the mean tangents of the teeth under examination.

Inter-proximal spaces and the coronal portions of the teeth may be secured perfectly on a roentgenogram by the use of any ordinarily used film if the simple method of Dr. Samuel J. Cohen be followed. It is attained merely by fastening an ordinary index tab, Dennison's No. 6, to the emulsion side of the film packet; and, in case the operator deems reinforcement of the tab necessary, by the addition of Dennison's gum reinforcement No. 17 pasted over it.

EXTRA–ORAL ROENTGENOLOGY.

Extra-oral roentgenograms are used for the examination of lesions of the jaws which cannot be obtained by the intra-oral methods. The roentgenologist must have a profound knowledge of the anatomical structures through which the rays pass before he attempts this type of examination.

The seven regions which may be examined by the extra-oral method are:

1. The mandible, from the canine region posterior to include the lower third of the ascending ramus.

2. The temporo-mandibular articulation.

3. The lateral aspect of the head.

4. The anterior-posterior view of the maxillary sinuses.

5. The anterior-posterior view of the frontal sinuses.

6. The superior view of the sphenoidal sinus.

7. The superior-inferior view of the malar bone and the zygomatic process.

1. The area involved in the first of this group must be carefully visualized as in Fig. 97. The cassette containing the film is then placed against the head-rest of the chair and allowed to rest on the patient's shoulder. The plane of the cassette should be approximately at an angle of 30 degrees from a perpendicular to the plane of the floor. The side of the head to be examined is then poised against and on the cassette in a position to ensure the malar bone and the chin touching the cassette. To maintain this position the head should be strapped to head-rest of the chair with a 2-inch bandage. (Fig. 98.) The tube is then placed in such a position as to have the direct rays parallel to the floor, *i. e.*, the vertical angle of the tube is 0 degrees and the the horizontal angle 90 degrees, the rays being centered over angle of the mandible nearest the tube. (Fig. 105.) This position will give the result as seen in Fig. 99.

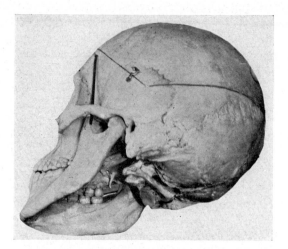

FIG. 97.—Area showing region to be examined. The operator must have a clear visualization of the anatomical structures through which the rays must pass before attempting any extra-oral roentgenogram of the mandibular third-molar region.

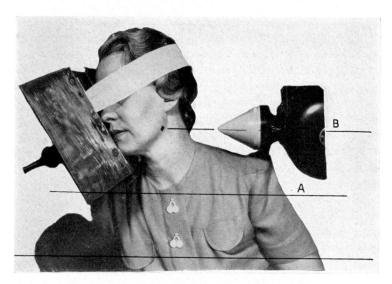

FIG. 98.—Relationship of the sagittal plane of the head to the plane of the film, the direct rays being parallel to the floor. This is the position to be maintained when examining the region shown in Fig. 97.

2. The area involved in the second of this group must be visualized as in Fig. 100, in which we now see the condyloid process of the ramus. The cassette is placed against the head-rest of the chair at an angle of 30 degrees from a perpendicular to the plane of the floor and resting on the patient's shoulder. The side of the face to be

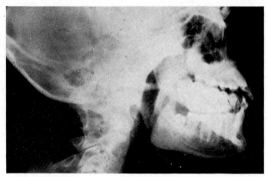

FIG. 99.—Extra-oral roentgenogram taken according to the technique shown in Fig. 98.

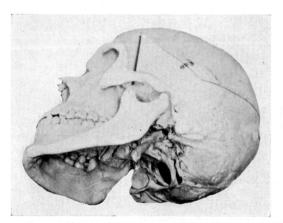

FIG. 100.—Area to be visualized clearly in the temporo-mandibular articulation.

examined is then placed on the cassette, the sagittal plane of the head being parallel with the mean plane of the cassette. (Fig. 102.) The head is extended forward in such a manner as to prevent the condyloid process from being superimposed over the vertebra of the neck (Figs. 101 and 104), and this position maintained by strapping the head to the head-rest by means of a 2-inch bandage. The tube is then set at 0 degrees in the vertical plane, and in the horizontal plane 5 degrees anteriorly from a perpendicular to the sagittal plane.

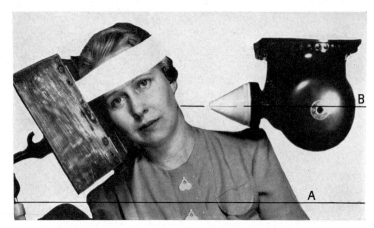

Fig. 101.—Relationship of the sagittal plane of the head to the plane of the film. (*B*) The direct rays parallel to the floor plane (*A*). This position to be maintained when examining the region shown in Fig. 100.

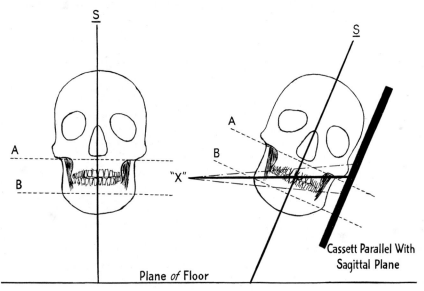

Fig. 102.—The method used to determine the lateral tilt of the head when making roentgenograms of the condyloid process.

The rays being centered over the angle of the mandible nearest the tube (Fig. 105), this position will give the result seen in Fig. 103. But, so that the lateral movement of the head of the condyle may be studied, and also the lateral displacement of the coronoid process

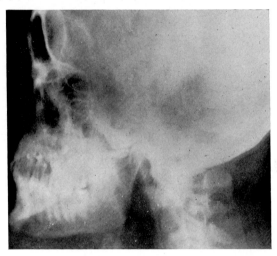

FIG. 103.—Extra-oral roentgenogram showing the result obtained by following the technique shown in Fig. 101.

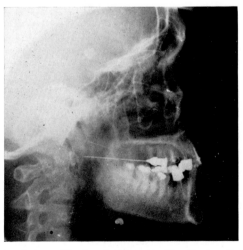

FIG. 104.—Lateral view of the head, demonstrating the localizing of a broken needle.

8

or of the condyloid process of the ramus following fractures of the condyle, we employ an additional or supplemental method of examination.

This is attained by placing the cassette containing the film parallel with the floor, placing the head of the patient on the cassette (Fig. 106), holding it in that position with a 2-inch bandage.

The rays are then directed perpendicular to the plane of occlusion, parallel with the sagittal plane, but through the temporo-mandib-

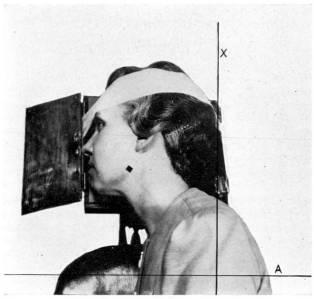

Fig. 105.—Point of entry of the central rays for lateral plates of the jaws. (*A*) plane of the floor; (*X*) the spine perpendicular to the plane of the floor, the head extended forward with the mean plane of the face perpendicular to the floor.

ular articulation and parallel to the posterior border of the ascending ramus, giving the result seen in Figs. 107 and 108.

3. The area involved in the third group is best taken with the head in the same relationship to the cassette as seen in Fig. 101, the central rays, however, being directed perpendicular to the sagittal plane of the head. This position gives the result seen in Fig. 104.

4. The area involving the maxillary sinuses is best recorded by placing the nose and chin of the patient on the cassette, with

the sagittal plane of the head perpendicular to the plane of the floor, the head being held in position by means of a 2-inch bandage. The tube is then placed in position, the central rays being directed along a line passing directly through the maxillary sinuses and paralleling the sagittal plane. (Fig. 109.) The best results are

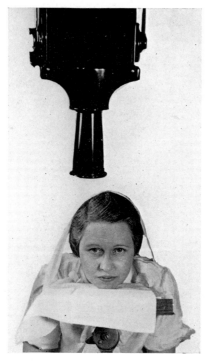

Fig. 106.—Position used when making a vertical view of the temporo-mandibular articulation, the head upon the cassette in the same position as used for making an examination of the sphenoid sinus (Figs. 112 and 113). The tube is shifted laterally so that the direct rays will pass through the sigmoid notch, as illustrated, giving the resultant roentgenograms as seen in Figs. 107 and 108.

obtained from a 36-inch target-plate distance. This, however, requires apparatus delivering a greater voltage than the average smaller dental unit provides. The result given is as seen in Fig. 110. With the small dental units, the target-plate distance is much shorter, and, therefore, the distortion is greater, as shown in Fig. 111. The shorter the target-plate distance, the greater is the amount of distortion. Comparing Fig. 110 with Fig. 111, which are roentgenograms of the same patient, one can readily note the distortion resulting from the decrease in the target-plate distance in addition to the difference in the size of the roentgenograms. But the operator must realize that the extra-oral method of examination alone is not sufficiently reliable to assure certainty of all appearances of abnormal or pathological conditions in the maxillary sinuses. It should be supplemented with intra-oral roentgenograms, the technique for which is suggested on pages 102, 103, 104 and 105.

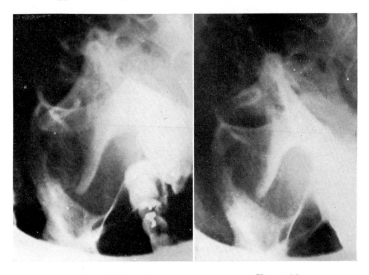

Fig. 107   Fig. 108

Fig. 107.—Roentgenogram of the temporo-mandibular articulation with the teeth in occlusion.

Fig. 108.—Roentgenogram of the same case as in Fig. 107 but patient has been instructed to open the mouth as far as possible, showing the condyloid process to have moved forward and slightly lateral to the position it assumed in Fig. 107.

5. The area involved in the fifth group, the frontal sinuses, is best recorded by placing the chin on the cassette, with the mean plane of the face 45 degrees to the plane of the cassette, the head being held in this position by means of a 2-inch bandage. The central rays are then directed along a line passing through the apex of the head to the superior border of the orbit and parallel to the sagittal plane. (Fig. 113.) Following the technique, one will obtain the result seen in Fig. 114.

6. Often enough, finding nothing in the roentgenograms indicating conditions to cause the trouble about which the patient complains, the operator resorts to making a roentgenologic study of the paranasal sinuses in an endeavor to ascertain if the trouble could have been created by some pathological condition pertaining to them. And while the area involved in this group presently discussed is not directly connected with the teeth, it is one of the paranasal sinuses, and, therefore, allied closely with the oral cavity.

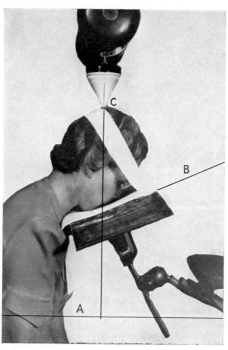

Fig. 109.—Relationship of the sagittal plane of the head to the plane of the film for the examination of the maxillary sinuses. (*A*) the central rays perpendicular to the floor and passing in a direct line through the sinuses; (*B*) the plane of the cassette twenty-three (23) degrees from the plane of the floor (*A*). The head is held firmly by means of a gauze bandage. The target-plate distance will vary with the type of equipment used. Direct rays follow line (*C*).

Owing to its position in relation to other anatomical structures of the head, it is necessary to use a technique differing from that used for other sinuses. But, and it depends upon the specific case

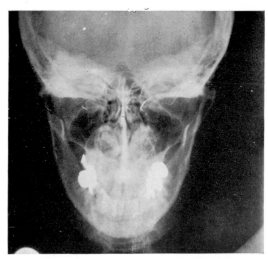

FIG. 110.—Extra-oral roentgenogram of the maxillary sinuses, using 36-inch target-plate distance, with apparatus equipped to supply a 5-inch back-up and 10 milliampères.

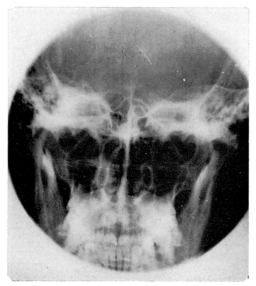

FIG. 111.—The same case as shown in Fig. 110, but at a target-plate distance of 20 inches. This distance was necessitated because an apparatus allowing only 3-inch back-up and 10 milliampères was used. Note the distortion, due to excessive divergence of the shadows of the object. Explanation in Fig. 112.

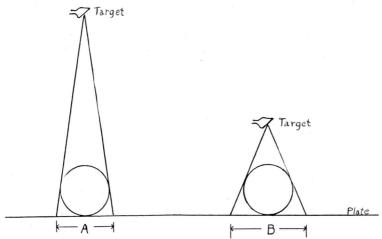

Fig. 112.—Illustrating the different size of shadow produced by varying the target-plate distance. The shorter the target-plate distance the greater the distortion. *A* represents conditions under which roentgenogram in Fig. 110 was produced. *B* represents conditions under which roentgenogram in Fig. 111 was produced.

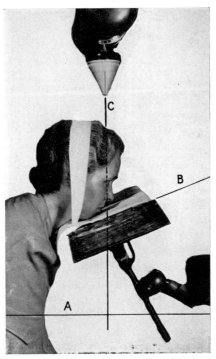

Fig. 113.—Relationship of the sagittal plane of the head to the plane of the film for examination of the frontal sinuses. The chin is placed upon the plate and the head retained in position by means of a gauze bandage. The direct rays following the line (*C*); the plane of the cassette (*B*) is twenty-three (23) degrees from the plane of the floor (*A*).

(119)

presented, we have a choice of methods of examination, the determining factor as to the technique employed being the length of the neck of the patient and the ability to extend the head so that it takes the position shown in Fig. 115.

So that with a patient having a long or an average size neck, the technique to follow is to place on a table the cassette holding

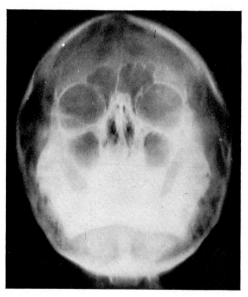

Fig. 114.—Extra-oral roentgenogram of the frontal sinuses, the result of following the technique demonstrated in Fig. 113.

the film in a position parallel with the floor, the patient being then placed in the position shown in the illustration. The edges of the cassette should touch the clavicle, with the patient's head extended to have the anterior surface of the neck and chin in contact with the casette, the mean plane of the head being as nearly perpendicular to the cassette as possible. The head is held in that position by a 2-inch bandage. (Fig. 115.)

The tube is angulated in a position anterior-posteriorly so as to have the direct rays parallel with the mean plane of the face, but on a line with the anterior border of the ascending ramus (Fig. 115) and horizontally through the center of the head parallel with the sagittal plane of the head. (Fig. 116.)

This will show the sphenoidal sinus between the right and left mandible. (Fig. 117.)

But if it prove impossible to follow the method explained because the patient has a neck too short to permit the extension required, good results may be obtained by placing the cassette as just sug-

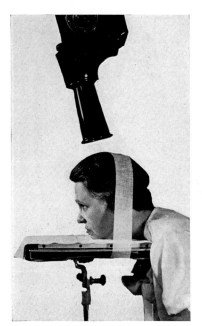 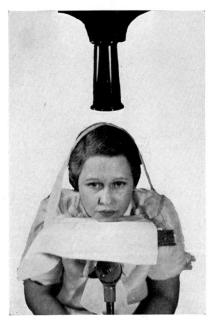

Fig. 115   Fig. 116

Fig. 115.—Head is placed on the cassette with the neck extended and held in place by a 2-inch bandage. The roentgen-rays are then directed downward paralleling the mean plane of the face, but passing through the apex of the head, about 2 cm. anterior of an imaginary line drawn between the right and left condyloid processes of the mandible. See result in Fig. 117.

Fig. 116.—The roentgen-rays must also parallel the sagittal plane of the head to give the result seen in Fig. 117.

gested, the head of the patient down, face upon the cassette, with the sagittal plane of the head perpendicular to the cassette. The patient is instructed to open his mouth as wide as possible. (Fig. 118.) To prevent movement, the head is held in position by a 2-inch bandage.

The tube is placed so that the direct rays will pass through the head, paralleling the sagittal plane on a line from the oral cavity through the temporo-mandibular articulation to the crest of the head. (Fig. 118.)

The sphenoidal sinus will then be seen superimposed over the oral cavity. (Fig. 119.)

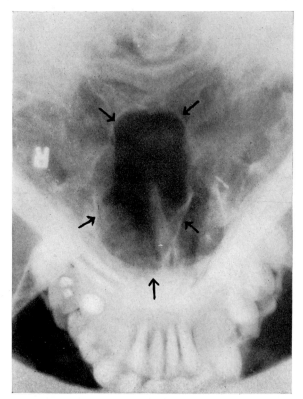

Fig. 117.—Roentgenogram the result of the technique shown in Figs. 115 and 116. The arrows point to the sphenoidal sinus.

7. Traumatic injuries to the head often involve the malar regions, and because of the location and the form of the malar bone and of the zygomatic process, a roentgenologic examination requires a definite technique that comprises the placing of the cassette in the position explained in paragraph 6 for examination of the sphenoidal sinus (Fig. 115), the head held immovable by a 2-inch bandage.

The tube is placed so that the direct rays will pass through the anterior portion of the head through the maxillary sinuses, parallel

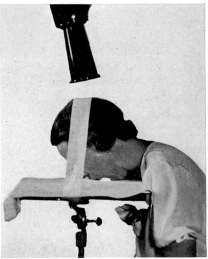

Fig. 118.—Face is placed upon the cassette with the mouth open as far as possible and the roentgen-rays directed through the apex of the head parallel with the sagittal plane and on an imaginary line passing through the temporo-mandibular articulation and the center of the oral cavity. The results may be seen in Fig. 119.

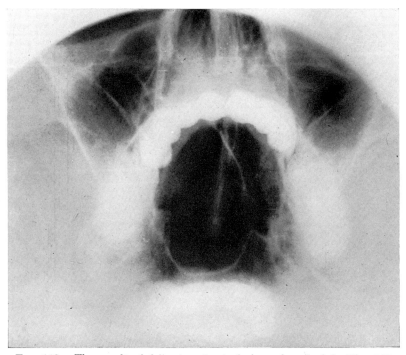

Fig. 119.—The result of following the technique described in Fig. 118. Note the sphenoidal sinus superimposed over the oral cavity.

(123)

with the face, perpendicular to the plane of occlusion, and parallel with the sagittal plane of the head.

The tube may be shifted to the right or left of the sagittal plane where a more detailed study of the injured part is necessary, giving a roentgenographic result as seen in Fig. 120.

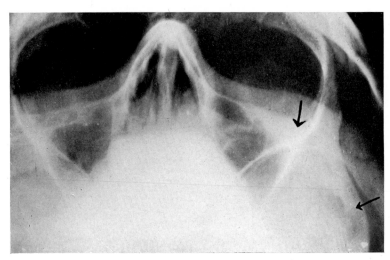

Fig. 120.—Roentgenogram revealing the zygomatic arch and malar process obtained by following technique described in Fig. 116, with the following exception: the rays are directed downward, paralleling the plane of the face and paralleling the sagittal plane.

THE PLACEMENT OF FILM IN THE ORAL CAVITY.

The placement of film should be accomplished with a facile deftness that connotes assurance and creates the impression that the operator has had long and experienced practice. Indecisive or clumsy insertions of the packets must be recognized by the patient whose inferences may be drawn to the discredit even of an outstandingly scientific roentgenologist; but ever so often we do meet with a dentist, and so with a roentgenologist, whose manual dexterity is not as high as the profession demands.

Necessary deftness may be acquired by practising the simplest method of film placement. Just as visualization of anatomical structures is essential before the position of the tube and the direction of rays for the exposure are determined, so is visualization of the position and the inclination of the teeth under observation essential before any attempt is made to insert film into the mouth of the patient. There is a technique in film placement that is very natural, very simple, and yet very precise, and by following it carefully an easy and assured dexterity must be achieved.

Maxillary Teeth.—For the maxillary molar region, the film should be held between the index finger and the thumb, and must be inserted horizontally into the mouth. Never, in handling the film for maxillary exposures, must it be bent or allowed in any way to become misshapen. To bend or twist the film before it is used may tend to take it out of a straight plane and may thereby produce distortions in the negative. The film packets come especially prepared to meet every ordinary requirement, and that includes a possible fine conformance with the anatomical lines and structures against which the film may be held.

Maxillary Molars.—For maxillary left molar teeth, the film, held between the thumb and index finger of the right hand, is passed into the mouth with the mean plane of the film packet parallel to the plane of occlusion and carried back until it reaches a position where the second molar is in the center of the outer margin of the film. Thereupon, the index finger of the left hand engages the outer margin of the film packet, the film resting parallel with the plane of occlusion and against the occlusal surface of the molars with the outer margin of the packet parallel to and extending to the buccal cusps of the molars. With the right index finger, the packet is rotated gently over the lingual cusps of the molars, and takes its final position against the soft tissues of the palate. The patient now assists by pressing his right thumb on the film against the coronal portion of the second molar, the fingers of his right hand naturally resting against the outside of his cheek to stabilize the position of his thumb and prevent movement of the film. (Fig. 52.)

To ascertain the relative position of the packet to the occlusal surfaces of the teeth, the operator may run his left index finger along the lower border of the film packet, which should be parallel with, but about ⅛ inch below, the occlusal surfaces of the molars. And the film should remain in practically a straight plane, the long axis of the teeth parallel with the short axis of the film.

Maxillary Left Premolars.—For the maxillary left premolars we follow the same steps as were covered in the case of the molars; only there is the natural exception that here the film must be so inserted and placed within the mouth that the premolars will contact with the center of the film, the long axis of the teeth paralleling the short axis of the film.

Maxillary Right Canine.—For the maxillary right canine, the film, its mean plane horizontal, is carried into the mouth and placed in a position so that the canine is in the center of the film and the long axis of the tooth will be parallel with the long axis of the film.

Maxillary Incisors.—For the maxillary incisors the film is carried into the mouth in a horizontal plane, the long axis of the film being placed in a position parallel with the long axis of the incisors.

Rules Guiding Placement of Film for Maxillary Teeth.—1. Avoid misshaping or bending film before inserting.

2. Carry film into the mouth by the thumb and index finger, holding the mean plane of the film parallel with the plane of occlusion.

3. Teeth under examination should be in the center of the film.

4. Maintain proper relationship between the long axis of the teeth and the long axis of the film.

5. Position the lower margin of the film approximately $\frac{1}{8}$ inch below the occlusal surfaces of the buccal margins of the teeth.

6. Patient holds film with thumb of hand opposite to side whereon operator is working, light pressure being exerted against the coronal portion.

7. Other fingers on the hand of patient, particularly the index finger, will rest against the side of his face, palm usually open, fingers extending perpendicular to plane of occlusion. (Fig. 55.)

Mandibular Teeth.—For roentgenograms of the mandibular teeth, never have the feeling that you must force the film into the proper position. It should be placed properly with the easiest gesture, the slightest pressure; and where any more pressure does seem called for it should be evident immediately that there are probably interposing conditions hindering the operator. These should be removed or corrected. Sometimes the lower anterior corner of the film packet may not have been turned sufficiently inward to escape tissue resistance; and in such a circumstance the packet should be withdrawn and the condition relieved by the further bending of the lower anterior corner of the film packet. Some patient may unconsciously oppose the operator by tensing the muscles in the floor of the mouth, thereby preventing the film from fitting into its proper position; and to overcome that condition the patient must be told to simulate swallowing, which relaxes the muscles and allows the film placement to proceed. Once the film is placed in the mouth, the patient will tolerate it without discomfort.

Mandibular Molars.—For roentgenographic examinations of the mandibular molars, the head of the patient having been tilted backward until the plane of occlusion is parallel with the plane of the floor, the film is held between the thumb and index finger. But before inserting it in the mouth, the operator should bend the lower anterior corner of the film slightly inward. This is a very distinguishing feature contrasting with the rules governing the careful handling of the film in the cases of the maxillary teeth; but for the mandible this step is taken so that, in the mouth, the bent corner will converge easily toward the sagittal plane.

The film packet is carried into the mouth and placed in a vertical position between the side of the tongue and the lingual surface of the teeth; and then the index finger of the other hand is placed against the back of the packet to maintain the position. With the index finger of the placing hand on the upper border of the film packet, and with easy pressure, the film should be moved backward and downward, so that the anterior border of the packet will be on a line with the inter-proximal space between the second premolar and the first molar. The upper border of the packet should be approximately 3 mm. above the occlusal surface of the teeth, and the long axis of the teeth parallel with the short axis of the packet. This position will assure a comprehending of the mandibular third molar and its roots even though it be impacted.

Once set properly, the film is held in position by the patient, whose index finger of the hand opposite the side under examination is placed against the back of the film packet; and, from the lateral pressure exerted against the film packet by the index finger in the region of the coronal portions of the teeth, the back or side of the hand of the patient will be resting against his face to add further support in maintaining the position of the film for the exposure. (Fig. 63.)

Mandibular Premolars.—In the mandibular premolar region the floor of the mouth is not as deep as it is in the molar region. So in preparing the film for insertion into the mouth we must bend the lower anterior corner of the film packet to a greater degree for roentgenograms of the mandibular premolar regions then we do for those of the molar region.

The packet, held between the thumb and the index finger, is so placed in the mouth that the long axis of the teeth parallels the short axis of the packet, the premolars in the center of the film. The packet is held in position by the index finger of the opposite hand touching against the back of it while the film is pressed lightly downward by the index finger of the first hand. This easy downward movement should proceed until the upper border of the film packet is 3 mm. above the occlusal surfaces of the premolars. Thereupon the index finger of the patient is placed upon the back of the packet, lateral pressure exerted against the coronal region, the side of patient's hand resting against the face affording further support to the stability of the position during exposure. (Fig. 63).

Mandibular Canines.— In the mandibular canine region the placing of films demands a particularly definite technique if longitudinal

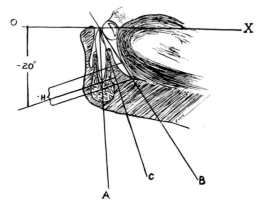

Fig. 121.—Illustrating the proper technique of holding the film in the anterior portion of the mandible. The pressure of the finger is upon the coronal portion of the tooth, allowing the film to remain in a straight line. Line *OX*, plane of occlusion; *A*, mean plane of the tooth; *B*, mean plane of the film; *C*, mean bisecting path at which rays must be directed; *H*, path of direct rays. Close adherence to this technique will prevent distortion of the apical portions of the teeth in this area.

distortions are to be prevented from appearing on the negatives. The film is bent along its long axis and placed in the mouth with the long axis of the film paralleling the long axis of the tooth, the lower border of the film against the frenum of the tongue, the upper border of the film about $\frac{1}{8}$ inch above the incisal margin of the tooth. With the index finger of patient touching the back of the film packet with pressure against the lingual surface of the canine, the film will remain in one plane, and the possibility of distortion eliminated or measurably decreased. (Fig. 121.) For distortion does so often result, especially where the apical third of the roots appear, when the film is held near the base and a bending along its short axis caused thereby. (Fig. 122.)

Guides for Placing of Film for Mandibular Teeth.—1. Distinguished from placements in the maxilla, for mandibular teeth the film packet must be bent before insertion.

2. Carry film into the mouth by thumb and forefinger.

3. Teeth under examination must be in the center of the film.

4. In the molar and premolar regions the long axis of the teeth should parallel the short axis of the film.

5. In the canine and incisor regions the long axis of the teeth should parallel the long axis of the film.

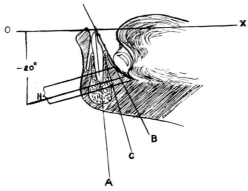

Fig. 122.—Illustrates how a film is bent when held in the mouth with the pressure of the finger exerted along the base of the film causing the film to bend backward in the floor of the mouth and so create distortion of the apical region when using a definite angulation.

6. Never force film into position. Either bend the film properly to conform, or, when met by resistance of patient, have him simulate swallowing.

7. Placement of film in the canine regions requires especially the maintenance of the packet in a straight plane on its long axis.

8. The index finger of the patient must be used as indicated to stabilize the position of the film during and just before exposure. (Fig. 63.)

Film-holders.—In addition to the manual method of holding the film in position by the thumb for exposures in the maxillary region and by the index finger for exposures of the mandibular teeth, there is the other method of placing the film packet on a small bite-block

9

film-holder (Fig. 72), which is inserted in the mouth and the patient instructed to hold in position by biting upon it.

An obvious advantage that would favor the manual method is the realization that, besides being efficient, its routine occupies the mind of the patient by affording an opportunity to assist in the procedure and serving to relieve the nervous tension found in many persons. But there are very apparent disadvantages inherent in the use of the holder; for the bite-block resting upon the teeth under examination, the film cannot extend far enough beyond the apical region to allow any latitude for examination of the apical tissues and structures. (Fig. 73.) More, the mouth closing upon the block prevents the operator from checking the position of the film with any assurance, for he sees almost no part of the mouth, a difficult barrier when attempting to angulate the tube to meet abnormal conditions. Thus many cases of exposures with the use of bite-block holder disclose distortions indicating elongations of the teeth examined.

Placement of the Occlusal Film.—The occlusal film, prepared particularly for the purpose of securing more general and comprehensive indications of possible pathological conditions in areas the smaller intra-oral film could not accommodate, allows fuller roentgenographic examinations of the maxilla, the mandible, or the floor of the mouth.

The emulsion is on one side only, it being easily observed as the one without folds, the smoother side of the packet.

During exposures, the emulsion side of the film must face the tube and the part of the oral cavity under examination. In examinations of the maxilla, the smooth side of the packet will face the palate; while in examinations of either the mandible or the floor of the mouth, the smooth surface of the packet, the emulsion, will face the tongue.

The corners of the red wax paper wrapping enveloping the film must be turned under, and the film inserted into the mouth parallel with the plane of occlusion and carried posteriorly as far as possible. Thereupon the film must be held in position by the patient biting upon it. (Fig. 81.)

GAGGING.

Every once in a while operators meet with patients whose reactions to the slightest pressure against the roof of the mouth and the palate result in gagging or even vomiting. These cases are usually met with in types of extremely nervous people or in cases of persons having really hypersensitive tissue in those regions. Of course, the difficulty is often overcome by a reassuring and smiling word from the operator. Yet, many cases refuse to react sufficiently under this simple plan.

Gagging is often attributable to the incorrect positioning of the head by the operator while attempting to insert the film packet, and very often it can be averted by seeing that the position of the head is so placed that the plane of occlusion is parallel with the plane of the floor.

Another common cause of gagging comes from the failure to instruct the patient as to the proper method of breathing; for it is not unusual for a patient to breathe through the mouth while holding the film in position with the thumb, the rush of air passing over the thumb causing irritation, however slight, to sensitive membranes. If the patient be instructed to hold the film with the thumb by exerting pressure against the lingual surface of the coronal third of the teeth, it will relieve the pressure of the film against the soft tissues to a great degree; and if the patient be advised to breathe through the nose, thus avoiding the rush of air over the sensitive tissues of the soft palate, the prospect of eliminating gagging may be fairly assured. The method also has the psychological effect of taking the mind of the nervous patient away from the procedure.

There may be extreme cases that refuse to respond to these easy remedies. An anesthesine calcidin troche (Abbott) dissolved on the tongue of the patient will produce a mild local anesthesia of the peripheral nerve endings and will cause no discomfort. It is not unpleasant, the palate becoming numb slowly, and the effects pass in about twenty minutes. This treatment will answer for the most stubborn cases.

CHAPTER IV.

ROENTGENOGRAPHIC EXAMINATIONS OF CHILDREN.

THE care of deciduous teeth should constitute the basic function of the dentist. To prevent premature loss is the primary problem, aiming toward preventive measures to avoid disease rather than to find later pathologic conditions requiring radical corrective treatment.

Deciduous teeth do become septic and create menaces to the health of children. (Fig. 123.) The longer the menace remains undetected the greater will be the insidious effect upon the mental and physical condition of the child. Too early loss (Fig. 124) or too long retention (Fig. 125) of deciduous teeth may result in irreparable destruction of normal occlusion and other vicious abnormalities (Fig. 126). Well hidden caries can be discovered only by early and continuous examinations (Fig. 127). Without thorough discovery, for which the roentgenogram is often our sole means, corrective measures cannot be taken intelligently.

Basic Problems.—To understand the basic problems in applying roentgenology to children, we must know the processes of calcification of both deciduous and permanent teeth; and we may notice calcification in the fetus at about the fifth month of intrauterine life, at which period we may observe a calcification of the incisors; (Fig. 128) and a progressive calcification is noticed from that period until the permanent third molar has calcified completely.

Calcification of Teeth.—At birth appears the first sign of calcification of the first permanent molar (Fig. 130), the cusps of the deciduous molars and canines have formed, the crowns of the deciduous incisors are fairly well developed, all of the teeth developing in bony crypts. It is with increasing calcium deposits during postnatal life that roentgenology becomes important in calculating the amount of development, for by obtaining thereby an appreciation of the rate of advance of the calcifying processes during early childhood we more accurately appraise our clinical findings; but when determining the amount of calcification of either deciduous or permanent teeth, it must be borne in mind that the marginal appearances of the developing teeth should be the main consideration rather than the appearance of the surfaces.

(132)

The roentgenogram disclosing information of a quantitative nature as to degree and stage of calcification, we may conclude as indications for treatment: (1) vitality and health of patient, (2) freedom

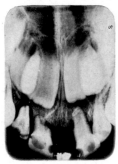
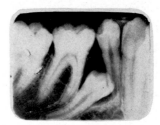

Fig. 123.   Fig. 124.

Fig. 123.—Deciduous maxillary incisors revealing a decided area of granulation tissue associated with absorption of the roots of the first incisors, also evidence of a suppurative condition around the left second incisor.

Fig. 124.—Early loss of the second deciduous molar causing the impaction of the second premolar due to a drifting of the molars.

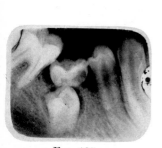
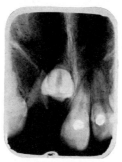
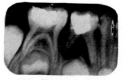

Fig. 125.   Fig. 126.   Fig. 127.

Fig. 125.—A depressed second deciduous molar locked in position by the first molar and first premolar causing a retention of the second premolar.

Fig. 126.—Deflection of the first incisior from its normal axial line, caused by too long retention of the deciduous teeth.

Fig. 127.—Small film made by cutting a regular intra-oral film in half. Reveals caries in both deciduous molars.

from systemic involvement, (3) degree of resorption, (4) tractability of the child, and (5) teeth where apices are closed and no necrotic tissue is present.

Similarly we deduce contraindications for treatment of deciduous teeth as (1) if more than one-third of the root is resorbed, (2) teeth with wide open apices due to destructive infective processes or necrotic tissues around the root, (3) where caries and infection have

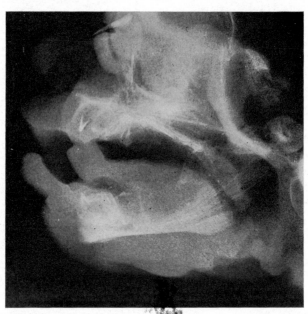

Fig. 128.—Roentgenogram of a fetus at five months revealing the developmental processes and centers of ossification of both the maxilla and mandible and the development of the maxillary incisors.

	Calcification begins								Calcification of the enamel completed and matured—crown fully formed.							
Upper	8	7	6	5	4	3	2	1	1	2	3	4	5	6	7	8
Lower	8	7	6	5	4	3	2	1	1	2	3	4	5	6	7	8
	7–10 yrs.	2½–3 yrs.	To 4 mo.	2–2½ yrs.	1½–2 yrs.	3–4 mo.	1 yr.	2–3 mo.	5 yrs.	5 yrs.	6 yrs.	6 yrs.	7 yrs.	3 yrs.	7 yrs.	? yrs.

Fig. 129.—Chart showing the calcification of the permanent teeth. (Kronfeld.)

destroyed the pulpal floor, and (4) where fistulas are present and open opposite free margins of the gums.

The crypts in which the teeth develop remain until the teeth erupt, when we observe the destruction of the crypt over the occlusal surface of the tooth; but we find the crypt about the tooth until the tooth is fully developed (Figs. 131 and 132). Misinterpretation of

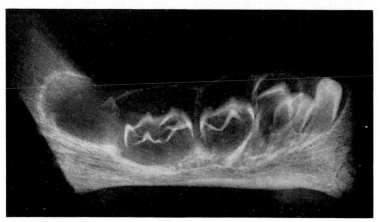

Fig. 130.—The development of the teeth at birth revealing the cusps of the first molar undergoing development and all teeth developing in bony crypts.

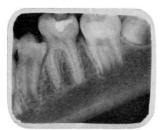   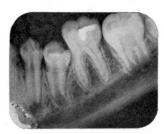

Fig. 131.   Fig. 132.

Fig. 131.—Crypt of the erupting mandibular second premolar superimposed on the first molar making the first molar appear as though absorbed.

Fig. 132.—Same case as Fig. 131 taken at a different angle, the crypt no longer superimposed.

the roentgenogram often results because the crypt partially surrounds the crown of the tooth until fully erupted; for at certain angles the roentgenogram may suggest a decalcification by reason of the crypt appearing superimposed over an adjoining tooth (Fig. 131), but changing the angulation of the tube will reveal the true condition if doubt exist. (Fig. 132.)

In cases where the ascending ramus raises very abruptly from the mandible these crypts sometime create a pocket, showing in the roentgenogram as a radiolucent area, thus presenting a condition preventing a complete eruption of the third molar. (Figs. 133, 134.)

Caries is more prevalent in childhood than in later life. During those years occur the greatest destruction and damage to teeth that

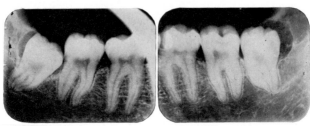

FIG. 133.   FIG. 134.

FIG. 133.—Developmental crypt of the third molar, often found when the ascending ramus rises abruptly from the mandible.

FIG. 134.—Right side of same case as Fig. 133 revealing the third molar in a vertical position, the crypt being much larger, probably developing into a dentigerous cyst, as seen in Fig. 590.

may continue to plague one throughout life, and it is essential that deciduous teeth be protected so as to function normally. It is a period when teeth are susceptible to good influences as well as to evil ones, a time for treatments to create a firmer structure to support advancing growth and to build resistance against future threats. There should be set up an immunity agains encroaching decay and disease, and immunity too often unattained until maturer years approach and avoidable ravages have done their damage. In both the preventive and restorative phases of dentistry roentgenology plays prominent rôles, especially with periodic examinations for lesions in their incipiency, caries especially, and to check on restorative work for indications of recurring lesions.

Caries existing at the earliest age of an infant, examination cannot be made too early if we would prevent malocclusion and other conditions we observe in the wake of caries. By discovering early trends of abnormalities (Fig. 135) the dentist provides against many physical disorders, mental sluggishness, defective eyesight and others, extending far beyond our province of ministrations but in meeting which dentistry can be of real aid.

We have for children the most complete dental clinics in the world. All are of comparatively recent pioneering incursions into the field hardly touched a few decades ago; but each succeeding day stresses their inestimable value and remind us how tardily medical science awoke to realize the part played by teeth of the youngest children in the health of a nation. The sinuses and more obvious abnormalities of the head were the visual indications of required treatment that were given attention when symptomatic conditions appeared; the hidden focus of infection that lurked in unerupted teeth and their surrounding structures remained too long unconsidered and unexplored.

There is no scientific difference in the general technique applied to the child and that applied to the adult. There may be a different

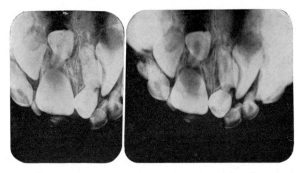

Fig. 135.—Supernumerary teeth causing the right first incisor to be rotated and the left first incisor to deviate from its normal axial line, child four years old.

approach because of the peculiar psychology of the patient, a distinction rarely appearing despite numerous mentions of it, but even then, as every dentist experiences, similarly varying conditions in adults demand varying approaches. Just as we observe different temperaments among individuals, there are different physical conditions to be considered. There are certain normal and certain peculiar factors in every patient. There are great variations in the sizes of anatomical structures of children just as there are wide differences between those of children and those of adults, and in making roengenographic examinations these differences require some deviation of procedure, usually a variation of the size of the intra-oral film or a method of placing the film to accommodate the condition met; but as to the proper relationship of the direct rays to the teeth and to the film, we always resort to the fundamental principles of roentgenology. The elimination of distortion is the goal, the principles governing the angulation for an adult control our technique for the child. With children both the intra-oral and extra-oral techniques are used, the choice depending upon the age and the parts under examination. To achieve the best results a combination of both techniques is generally the better procedure, for valuable information about the development of teeth and jaws can be secured with the extra-oral plates.

Age at Which Examinations are Made.—The highly important point in treatment of children concerns the age or period when such examinations should be made. This is a problem for which there is no simple answer. Whatever advice he would give, both as to the time and as to the importance of examinations and treatments, the dentist must first convince the parents of the necessity, and that is sometimes a difficult task. Until education takes larger strides toward enforcing a more intimate knowledge of the power of preventive measures in matters of health there will come no pressing demand on dentists to examine the oral cavities of infants. We examine the teeth of children when they are brought to us, and they are brought to us too seldom during the years when deciduous teeth become loose, to be pulled out by the same method our country cousins used sixty years ago: the piece of string, the doorknob, the sudden opening of the door, and then the wide open spaces disfiguring the child. No notion of maintaining the proper interstitial spaces between the temporary teeth to permit the natural eruption and growth of the permanents; no consideration of possible malformations that often follow improperly manipulated extractions. And in our present generation hardly more thought is given similar conditions; for while the string and the doorknob may be partially discarded methods, there still is no deep realization of the danger risked by inattention to the deciduous and to the early permanent teeth. Education of the parents is the sole solution of such a problem. Mothers must be taught that just as vaccination protects against future fevers and other illness, early roentgenographic examinations and indicated treatments of the child insures against future disfigurations, against too early edentulosity, against focal infections to disturb the systemic condition of the child.

Let routine examinations begin when the child is between three and four years of age, with exceptions for earlier observations when justified by accidents (Fig. 136) or other anomalous circumstances (Figs. 137, 138, 139, 140). Extra-oral plates for the right and the left sides (Figs. 141 and 142), and taking occlusal views of the maxillary anteriors (Figs. 135 and 143) would reveal the developmental processes of the teeth and jaws (Fig. 135), basic information upon which depends your deductions as to what treatments or the forbearance of them should follow. It is the time of the most important relationship between the deciduous and the developing permanent teeth, the period to prepare for eruption of the permanent molars; for too often these permanent molars are thought to have a natural later

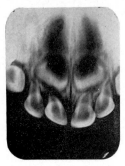

Fig. 136.—Case of child two years old having fallen and injured the anterior teeth, roentgenogram revealing the left maxillary first incisor deviating from its normal axial line.

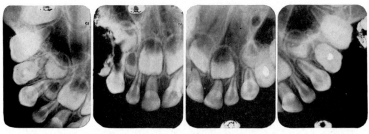

Fig. 137.   Fig. 138.   Fig. 139.   Fig. 140.

Figs. 137, 138, 139, and 140.—Examination of the maxilla of a three year old child using occlusal technique. Normal development is taking place except for the absence of the right second permanent incisor, the permanent left second incisor being in place.

replacement. The permanent first molar should be extracted only when corrective measures are inapplicable if we would avoid a threat of malformation that is not uncommon. That lesson should be read to all prospective mothers who really prepare for the health of the baby she awaits; for there are books about clothing, feeding,

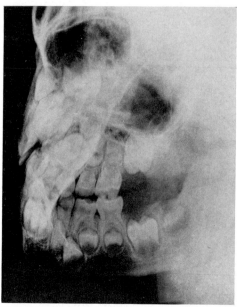

Fig. 141.—Lateral plate of a child four years of age revealing the developmental process taking place.   This type of exposure affords a greater knowledge than could be secured with intra-oral films.

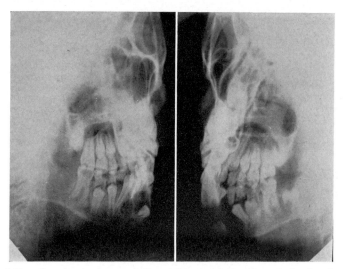

Fig. 142.—Roentgenograms of the right and left sides of the head of a child revealing both the mandible and the maxilla.

bathing and general hygiene, and as one of the leading topics of such books should be included full and illuminating advice about the care of the oral cavity and of the teeth though it be months before signs of the first one erupting appear.

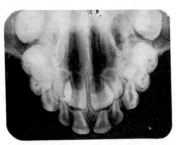

Fig. 143.—Occlusal view of a child three and one-half years old revealing developmental processes of maxillary anterior teeth.

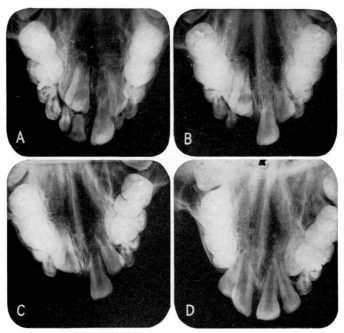

Fig. 144.—(*A*), A supernumerary tooth preventing the eruption of the left 1st incisor. The right 1st incisor has erupted. The left deciduous teeth are still in position; (*B*), deciduous teeth removed as suspected cause of the retention; (*C*), supernumerary tooth removed; (*D*), six months elapsed time. The incisors have erupted without mechanical aid.

Were women advised about this by the obstetrician there would be much less resistance to roentgenographic examinations later, at six, (Figs 141, 142, 148), say, and again at nine (Fig. 144) and twelve

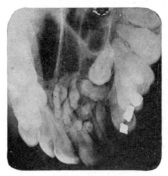 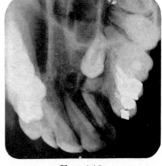

| Fig. 145. | Fig. 146. |

Fig. 145.—A segregate odontome in a fourteen year old child containing approximately twenty separate anomalous teeth.

Fig. 146.—Same case as Fig. 145, five months after operation. Reveals three anomalous teeth the operator failed to observe at the time of operation and stresses the necessity of making a roentgenographic examination immediately after operation.

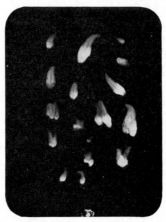

Fig. 147.—Anomalous teeth removed from the case shown in Fig. 145.

years of age (Figs. 145, 146 and 147), when the developmental phases of both normal or abnormal conditions are greatest. Each subsequent examination would find the intraoral technique more easily applied. No set rule should be enunciated as to the number of films used in the full-mouth examination of a child. The operator must determine that procedure as governed by the patient under treatment, the results confirming or denying his technique; for the end being a thorough examination of both teeth and surrounding structures, the number of films that assure this result must be used.

Any well prepared operator should be as capable of treating a child of six as he is of treating a grandfather of sixty years. The posted practitioners understand the anatomy of the maxilla, the mandible, the teeth and enveloping tissues of both sire and son, for otherwise they had better revert to some serious post-graduate study to learn anew some of the courses which their license to practice assumed they knew. If essential knowledge of any part of the oral cavity from the anatomical and pathological points of view be lacking, what

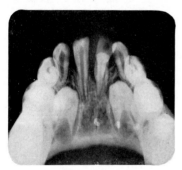 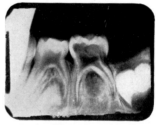

Fig. 148.	Fig. 149.

Fig. 148.—A retained deciduous incisor causing the mandibular first incisor to be forced from its normal axial line into the lip. There is also a congenital absence of the mandibular second incisors.

Fig. 149.—Chronic perforating hyperplasia of the pulp of the second deciduous molar.

dependence upon diagnoses, what reliance upon prognoses of the dentist? There is no tempering of responsibility for accuracy in dental ministrations, and to a child least of all.

Objective of Periodic Examination.—The objectives of periodic roentgenological examinations demand accuracy, for by them may be determined the absolute guide posts for treatment. We discover the time of calcification of each deciduous and permanent tooth, (Figs. 128, 130, 141), the divergence of deciduous molar roots (Fig. 149), and the anatomical characteristics of both deciduous and permanent teeth; we determine the time for removing deciduous teeth to permit the natural development of the jaws, and to provide against drifting of permanent teeth already erupting (Fig. 150), a condition creative of impactions and malocclusions that are not so uncommon in the mandibular and maxillary second premolar and maxillary canine regions (Figs. 151, 152, 153, 154, 155, 156, 157); and we

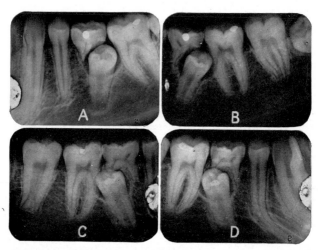

Fig. 150.—Revealing too long retention of deciduous second molar. (*A*) and (*B*) are the same case taken at different angles. (*C*) and (*D*) fall in the same category, both cases revealing a variation of the second premolar due to angulation.

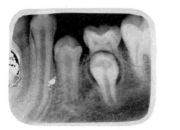

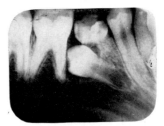

Fig. 151.   Fig. 152.

Fig. 151.—Revealing the second mandibular premolar inclined lingually from its normal axial line.

Fig. 152.—Mandibular second premolar with a distal angular inclination due to a too long retention of the deciduous teeth.

determine as well the reason for any relatively prolonged retentions of deciduous teeth. (Figs. 125, 144, 158.) In no other way could we find surely the amount of root resorption of deciduous teeth

(Fig. 159) or discover with near exactness the presence of super-numerary teeth, especially in the region of the maxillary incisors (Figs. 160 to 165); and the presence of supernumary teeth in the

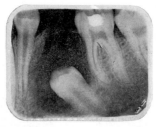

Fig. 153.—Dentigerous cyst involving the mandibular second premolar.

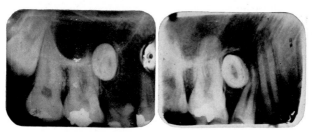

FIG. 154.   FIG. 155.

FIGS. 154, 155.—Too early loss of deciduous teeth, causing transversal impactions of the maxillary second premolars.

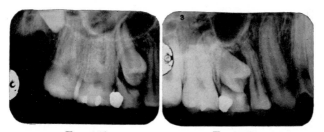

FIG. 156.   FIG. 157.

FIGS. 156, 157.—Too long retention of the second deciduous molar, causing the second premolar to deviate from its normal axial line.

maxilla is more common than realized, often causing the maxillary incisors to shift from the normal axial line (Fig. 164), or to rotate (Fig. 163), or to be retained beyond normality (Fig. 144). The roentgenogram will show any overhanging fillings (Fig. 166), and

10

it will disclose caries on proximal surfaces (Fig. 127), a most important service, for deciduous molars have broad contracting surfaces, making difficult detection of small proximal cavities; it will determine the presence of or congenital absence of the permanent teeth before they erupt and inform whether any absence is unilateral or bilateral.

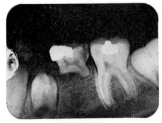
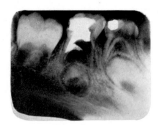

Fig. 158.   Fig. 159.

Fig. 158.—Retention of the second deciduous molar and congenital absence of the second premolar.

Fig. 159.—Partial absorption of the roots of second deciduous molar, revealing a perforation of the distal root and considerable loss of bone.

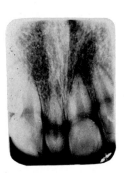
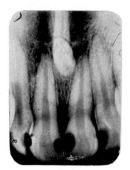

Fig. 160.   Fig. 161.

Fig. 160.—Supernumerary tooth erupted between the crowns of the first incisors.

Fig. 161.—Supernumerary tooth impacted between the roots of the first incisors in the apical region.

(Figs. 137 to 140, 169, 175.) The amount of pulp involvement (Fig. 149), the amount of alveolar loss due to infection (Figs. 167, 168), or the presence of residual deciduous roots should be indicated in the roentgenogram; and no substituted examination can reveal the amount of damage resulting from traumatic injury, for no treatment in such cases should ever be attempted without the knowledge afforded by a roentgenographic examination. (Fig. 136.)

Enumerating fully the possibilities of roentgenographic examinations would require a longer list than that presented. (Figs. 170, 171, 172.) We are discovering daily more and more disclosures on the roentgenogram that allow diagnoses and permit interpretations

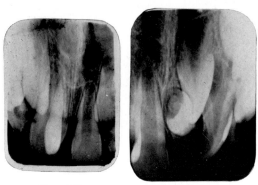

Fig. 162.   Fig. 163.

Fig. 162.—Supernumerary tooth erupted and forcing the left first incisor from its normal axial line. In the roentgenogram it appears superimposed over the first incisor.

Fig. 163.—Supernumerary tooth causing a rotation of the right first incisor.

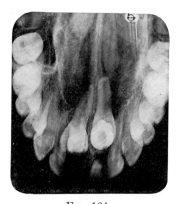 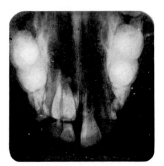

Fig. 164.   Fig. 165.

Fig. 164.—Two supernumerary teeth preventing the eruption of the two first incisors, the second incisors having completely erupted.

Fig. 165.—A supernumerary tooth preventing the eruption of the maxillary first incisor.

of conditions that had been merest guesses before. Peculiarly, it has been the findings of general practitioners that have led to the greatest realization of the powers of roentgenology; for whether at

first capable of interpreting the revelations or not, in the search
to find the meaning of strangely appearing areas that will crop up
out of the millions of roentgenograms taken, there has been given to
dentistry some of the highest knowledge of both anatomy and pathol-

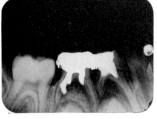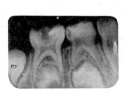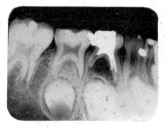

Fig. 166.   Fig. 167.   Fig. 168.

Fig. 166.—Attempted root canal filling of the deciduous molars, revealing perforated root of the second deciduous molar.

Fig. 167.—Small film No. 0 revealing an absorbed root of first deciduous
molar. Radiolucent area denotes a loss of bone under the same tooth due
to infection.

Fig. 168.—Showing extensive destruction of bone between the root of
the second deciduous molar and the crown of the developing premolar, due
to infection.

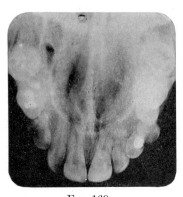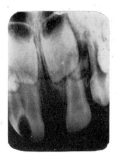

Fig. 169.   Fig. 170.

Fig. 169.—Congenital absence of the right and left maxillary canines.

Fig. 170.—False gemination of the deciduous maxillary first and second
incisors.

ogy. The knowledge gained from examinations of children of all
ages has widened enormously the field of dentistry.

Intra-oral Technique.—The best intra-oral roentgenography resulting from full coöperation of the patient, a very essential aid with
children, it is always better to have the patient hold the film.

(Fig. 174.) It produces confidence in the child, for to young patients a roentgenographic examination is a new experiment and gaining

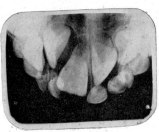 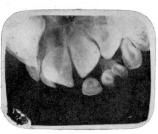 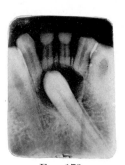

Fig. 171.   Fig. 172.   Fig. 173.

Figs. 171 and 172.—False gemination of the deciduous right first and second incisors deviating from their normal axial lines, resulting in a contraction of the maxilla and a deviation of the permanent incisors.

Fig. 173.—Congenital absence of the four mandibular incisors and a dentigerous cyst involving the mandibular permanent canine.

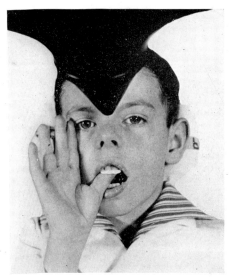

Fig. 174.—Position of child's head and hand when examining maxillary anterior teeth.

their confidence will make application of whatever technique used much easier.

When we speak of the age of a child, considered with the extent

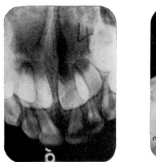 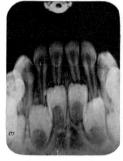 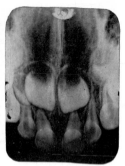

FIG. 175.   FIG. 176.   FIG. 177.

FIG. 175.—Normal development of the maxillary teeth at the age of four years.

FIG. 176.—Normal development of the mandibular teeth at the age of four years.

FIG. 177.—The congenital absence of the permanent right maxillary second incisor, the permanent left second incisor in place, at age of three and one-half years.

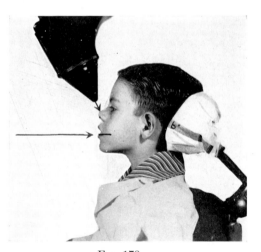

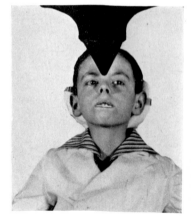

FIG. 178.   FIG. 179.

FIG. 178.—Position of the head of a child when making occlusal views or using a small film in the occlusal position to obtain the results seen in Figs. 143 or 177.

FIG. 179.—Position of head in relation to tube for roentgenograms of the anterior teeth in children, the plane of occlusion parallel with floor, the central rays parallel with the sagittal plane.

and purpose of the examination, in determining the type of film to be used, we must consider particularly the extent, the size, and the

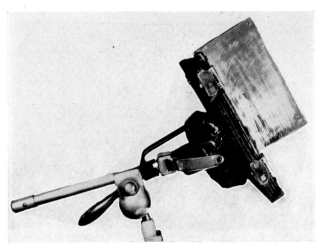

Fig. 180.—Simplified cassette holder for lateral plates of the jaws, showing the method by which it may be attached to and held rigidly to the head-rest of the dental chair.

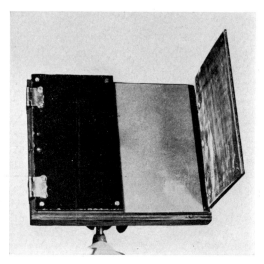

Fig. 181.—Front view of the cassette holder with the two lead screens one open and the other closed, enabling operator to take the right and left sides of the head on the same plate as revealed in Fig. 142.

developed growth of the oral cavity. We may assume that in a child from birth to six years, the preschool age, we would use a smaller film than those generally used. To meet individual requirements it

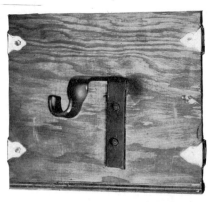

FIG. 182.—Back view of cassette holder showing the attachment apparatus which fastens the holder to the head-rest.

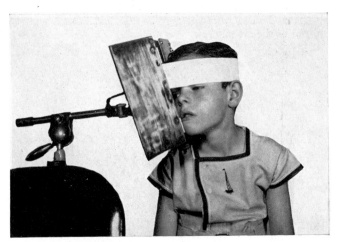

FIG. 183.—Correct position of the head and its relationship to the cassette holder where it is impossible to have patient sit in the chair. The use of the cassette holder prevents bending of the cardboard holder and gives stability.

may become necessary to cut a regular-sized film to a smaller dimension. (Fig. 127.) This is done in the dark room where the free edges are covered with adhesive tape to make it light proof. Of course smaller film packets are distributed by several film manufacturers. (Fig. 167.)

Consider the type of film suggested in the examination of a two year old child who has fallen and has depressed the maxillary incisors, probably one of the most difficult cases we meet. The injured child is apprehensive and harbors the animal instinct to be alone. To make a successful examination with the least discomfort to the patient we select a regular intraoral film, place it in the plane of occlusion, and have the patient bite upon the packet. (Figs. 178, 179.) Thus we employ the intra-oral film as an occlusal film to bring the results as seen in Figs. 136, 137 to 140, 175, 176, 177.

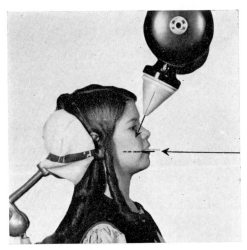

Fig. 184.—Position of head of child for an occlusal view of entire palate with the result seen in Fig. 144. Note rays passing through the upper third of nose.

Extra-oral Technique.—Further examinations of younger children becoming necessary, the lateral plate or the extra-oral method is advised, probably with the Eastman 8 x 10 inch No-Screen or the Afga Non-Screen film in the Eastman cardboard film holder, upon which both the right side and the left side of the oral cavity may be shown; for this result may be obtained by placing over one half of the film holder a piece of lead, approximately 4 x 5 x $\frac{1}{8}$ inches, and making an exposure on the side not so covered by the lead; then remove the lead, cover with it the other half of the film holder, exposing the other side of the oral cavity on the uncovered side of the film holder. (Figs. 180, 183.) This permits development of the two exposures in one treatment, and the both sides of the oral cavity appearing on the one film makes easier the comparison of the one side to the other. (Fig. 142.) Larger intra-oral films being used

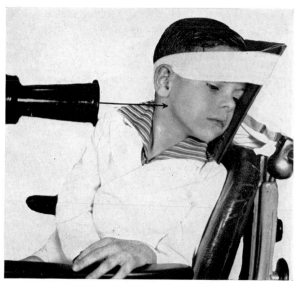

Fig. 185.—Correct position of the body and the head of a child and proper relationship of the central rays to the head and cassette. Note the maintenance of the head in position by the use of a bandage.

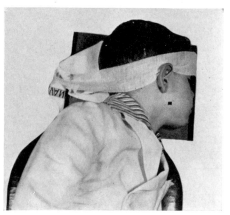

Fig. 186.—Front view showing the head extending forward and the shoulder back so as not to interfere with the radiation.

as a child grows older, with the greater development of the child regular intra-oral films will be used successfully, with regular occlusal film to obtain a general view of the maxilla. (Figs. 145 to 147, 184.)

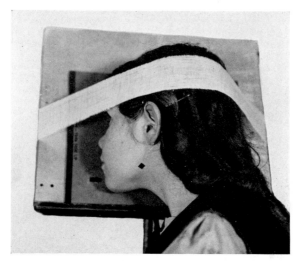

Fig. 187.—Position of head when making lateral roentgenograms of jaws; the body of the child in an erect position, head extended forward, the mean plane of the face parallel with the side of cassette.

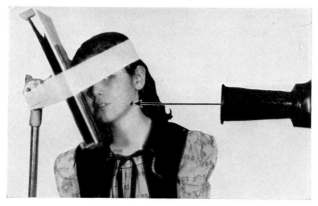

Fig. 188.—Side view of same technique explained in Fig. 187. Note position of the shoulder, which is completely out of the line of radiation.

The extra-oral technique of exposure may be done in a dental chair (Figs. 185, 186) or by employing a special head-rest separate from the chair. (Figs. 180, 181, 187, 188, 189.) The basic principle of the two methods is the same: If the chair is used, the patient sits upright in the chair, and sideways; the shoulders of the patient are back, the spinal column erect; the head-rest of the chair is tilted so that when the cassette is placed against it and rests against the shoulder of the patient, the cassette will be at an angle of thirty (30) degrees from a perpendicular to the floor. The head of patient is then extended as in craning the neck (Figs 186, 187), the face rotated toward the cassette until the long body of the mandible is in contact

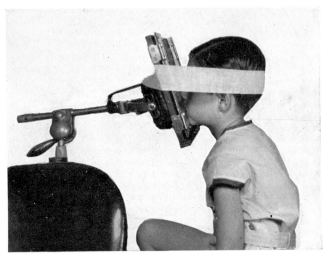

Fig. 189.—Position of the head and cassette holder when making sinus examination.

with the cassette, the tip of the nose almost touching it. (Figs. 185, 188.) If the child be not in proper position, the shoulder will interfere with placing the tube in proper relationship to the cassette; but once this correct position has been assumed, the tube is adjusted so that the central rays are parallel with the floor and directed at the angle of the jaw nearest the tube. (Figs. 185, 188.) The result is shown in Figs. 141, 142.

In making lateral roentgenograms of the jaw it is important to bind the head to the cassette with a bandage so as to immobilize the head and thus prevent the resultant image from being blurred by any movement during exposure. (Figs. 187, 188.) Considering in general the placement of film for a child patient, the same technique we use for an adult may be applied, but for the child of preschool age the best results are obtained with the extra-oral film for the posterior teeth, allowing the child to hold the film by biting upon it. (Fig. 179.) The result may be seen in Figs. 136 to 140. For older children the intra-oral examination is more common, the same technique as applied to adults being used.

Complications may arise when placing the film in the mandibular molar and premolar regions, for usually the floor of the mouth may not be very deep, or the patient may tend to contract the muscles in the floor of the mouth to create a similar condition; but this difficulty may be overcome by inserting the film into the mouth until meeting resisting tissues, whereupon the patient is coached to close his mouth until only his index finger may pass between the teeth, the index finger being used to hold the film in position. This procedure causes the muscles of the floor of the mouth to relax and thus permit the film to have a proper position without discomfort to the patient.

With intra-oral roentgenograms, children tend to rotate the head backward and thereby tense the muscles in the floor of the mouth. This may be avoided by having the child in the chair so that the long axis of the body approximates a perpendicular to the floor, the head-rest so adjusted as to prevent the child from tilting the head too far backward. This permits placement of the film more easily.

CHAPTER V.

METHODS OF LOCALIZATION.

STEREOROENTGENOGRAPHY.

This method of examination is not new; it was first suggested by Elihu Thompson, in 1896, and sometime later Sir James Mackenzie Davidson, of London, further developed the idea, and it has been employed in the medical field by roentgenologists since that time.

Only recently, however, the dental profession began using this means of examination. Ivy was one of the first to mention the importance of the proper use of stereoroentgenograms in diagnoses, but it is highly necessary to emphasize that the value depends on perfect technique and understanding. He was followed by Le Masters, who declares: "It has been grossly underestimated by some, and correspondingly exaggerated by others."

The principle of stereoroentgenography is valuable in that it adds perspective, or depth, to the roentgenogram.

Le Masters further suggests that: "The failure of the dental roentgenologist to use this method of examination extensively may be summed up as follows:

"1. The difficulty of placing two films accurately in the same position in the mouth for two exposures.

"2. Securing absolute immobilization of the patient between exposures.

"3. Determining the proper angles of the central rays with the two shifts of the tube.

"4. The proper mounting in the stereoscope.

"5. The difficulty experienced by some individuals in viewing stereoscopic films."

However reasonable these views might have been but a few years ago, the majority of those conditions have been overcome. Let us consider them in their order:

1. When necessity requires the placing of two films in the mouth in the same position for two exposures, we meet the condition by the use of metal film-holders.

There are two types of holders: one for the small dental film (Fig. 191) and the other for the bite film Eastman occlusal (Fig. 192).

(158)

For the small dental film the technique follows:

A small strip of modeling compound is placed on the occlusal rest of the film-holder; a film is then placed in the holder, the compound having previously been heated; the film and holder are now placed in the mouth, the soft compound coming in contact with the occlusal surface of the teeth and causing an imprint of the teeth to be made in the compound.

The metal film-holder prevents the film from bending, therefore succeeding films will be in the same plane. The first exposure is made, and the film and holder withdrawn. A second film is inserted into the holder, which is thereupon placed in the mouth in exactly

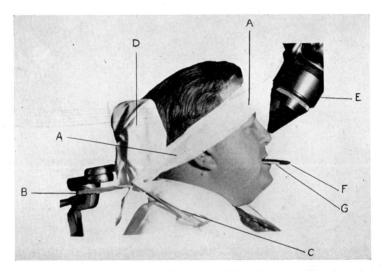

FIG. 190.—Illustrating the technique used for the immobilization of the head in taking stereoroentgenograms and for purposes of any other localization: *A*, a 2-inch gauze bandage placed around the forehead, passing back around the head-rest lock (*B*) and held together by means of a hemostat (*C*); *D*, the head-rest, with the head placed within it so that the occlusal plane is parallel to the floor; *F*, Eastman occlusal film placed in a film-holder (*G*), which is held between the occlusal surfaces of the teeth parallel to the floor; *E*, tube in position.

the same position as was the first film, a position assured because the teeth will slide into the impressions made in the compound at the time of the first exposure. Moreover, if desired, the small strip of compound may be removed and filed in order that the exact position may be attained at any futher date.

For the Eastman occlusal film, the bite film, the holder is of different design. It is so constructed that the film will slide in or out without coming in contact with the teeth. It has grooves on both sides and at the back in which the film fits. The film-holder is placed in the mouth in the bite position, the occlusal surfaces of the teeth coming in contact with the top of the grooves and thus re-

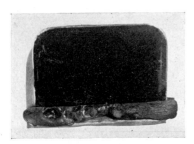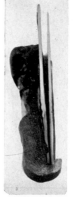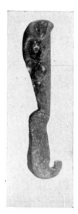

FIG. 191.—Film in holder, with modeling compound in position for stereo-scopic films. Same may be used for reproduction of roentgenograms.

taining the film-holder in a rigid position. Any number of films may now be placed consecutively in the mouth accurately and in the same position.

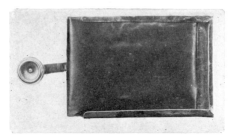

FIG. 192.—Film-holder for Eastman occlusal film, with film in position and with the spirit-level attached.

2. Immobilization of the patient between exposures may be obtained in a very simple manner. This is done by passing around the forehead of the patient a piece of 2-inch gauze bandage, extending it backward around the head-rest of the chair and clamping it with a hemostat. This prevents the patient from moving the head out of position. (Fig. 190.)

3. The determining angle of the central ray with the two shifts of the tube is: The tube is first centered over the part to be taken, and then shifted $1\frac{1}{4}$ inches to the right; it is then tilted in such a manner that the direct rays will pass through the same point of entry as they would pass if the tube were centered. The exposure is now made. The tube is, thereupon, moved back to the center, then shifted $1\frac{1}{4}$ inches to the left, where a similar procedure to that taken on the right side is followed. It will be observed that the tube has thus moved from right to left a total distance of $2\frac{1}{2}$ inches, corresponding to the distance between the pupils of the normal eyes. The angle of inclination of these rays will be $7\frac{1}{2}$ degrees toward the point of entry.

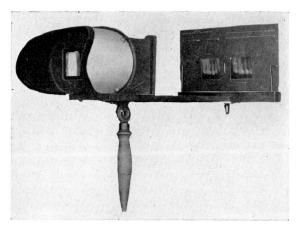

Fig. 193.—The ordinary hand stereoscope is well adapted for the purpose of viewing stereoroentgenograms.

4. The two films must be mounted in the stereoscope in a manner so that upon view they will blend into one. The essential point is that the films should take their proper places in the stereoscope— the right exposure on the right side and the left exposure on the left side of the stereoscope. If this detail be met, the results should be satisfactory.

5. Just as some individuals are color-blind, or astigmatic, so some persons have an eye fault anatomically antagonizing a proper stereoscopic illusion. That condition cannot be corrected by general advice; but an operator suffering any such shortcomings must be careful on his attempts at interpretation.

11

Method of Exposure.—*Summary.*—The patient's head is placed in the head-rest of the chair and adjusted until the various planes are in their proper position. The head is then secured, as in Fig. 190, to prevent movement, the film-holder with film placed in the mouth, and the roentgen-ray tube is brought to a position in which it would be placed for a normal exposure. This is known as centering. The tube being centered, it is then shifted $1\frac{1}{4}$ inches to the right, and

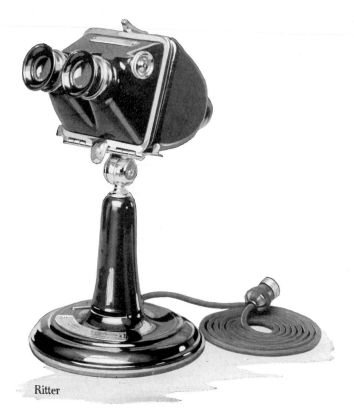

Fig. 194.—Later type, combining the principle of the stereoscope with a system of variable illumination for examining films of different density.

the first exposure is made. The film-holder and film are removed. A second film is placed in the holder, which is now returned to the mouth. The imprints of the teeth in the compound will allow the holder to assume its former position. The tube is now returned to center position, and then shifted $1\frac{1}{4}$ inches to the left, whereupon a second exposure is made. The films should be marked right and left and placed in the stereoscope in their proper position.

The *Clark technique* for the localization of impacted teeth involves a simple principle: Given two objects in a perfectly straight line with the observer, the more distant object will be hidden from sight by the other. If the observer moves to the right, the more distant object will apparently move to the right. Similarly, if the observer moves to the left, the more distant object will apparently move to the left. And as the more distant object seems to move toward the direction taken by the observer, the nearer object seems to move in the opposite direction. (Fig. 195.)

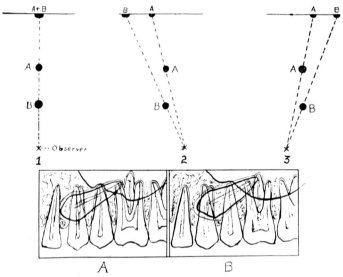

Fig. 195.—1. Two objects in a straight line with the observer; the more distant one is covered by the nearer. 2. Observer moves to the right; the more distant object is apparently to the right of the nearer one. 3. Observer moves to the left; the nearer object is apparently to the right of the more distant one. (Ivy.) *A*. Tip of canine touches the second incisor. *B*. Tube is moved to the right; the tip of the canine has moved away from the incisor and in the same direction as the tube; the canine is, therefore, the more distant object and lies on the lingual side.

Applying this principle to roentgenography, it is necessary to take two roentgenograms in the following manner: The patient's head is placed in the head-rest of the chair with the sagittal plane perpendicular to the floor and the plane of occlusion parallel to the floor; a film is then placed in the region of the mouth to be examined.

Either a small dental film or an Eastman occlusal film may be used, depending upon the area under examination. The tube is then placed in position, the film exposed, and marked exposure No. "1." A second film is then placed in the mouth in the identical position as was the first film, the planes of the head remaining the same.

Before the second exposure, the tube, while being allowed to remain in at the same vertical and horizontal angles employed in first exposure, is shifted approximately 2 cm. anteriorly or posteriorly, as the particular case demands. The direction of the shift will depend, of course, upon the relation between the tube and the area under observation when making the first exposure.

Taking two roentgenograms by this method, one from a position a little farther to the right of the other, we should be able to localize the condition existing.

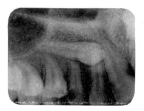 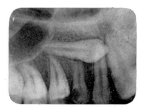

Fig. 196   Fig. 197

FIGS. 196 and 197.—Localized impacted teeth with small dental film. Fig. 196, showing canine tip touching shadow of the pulp of the first incisor. Fig. 197, tube moved distally, the tip of the canine is a considerable distance distal to the pulp of the first incisor, *i. e.*, the canine moved in the same direction as the tube; therefore, it is at a greater distance from the tube than the other teeth, and, hence, on the lingual side.

Comparing two roentgenograms so taken, we must determine whether our observation notes an unerupted tooth. If it does, our next step is to determine whether it be buccally or lingually situated.

If the unerupted tooth shows on the second film farther to the right than it appears on the first film, apparently it has moved in the direction of the shifted tube; and, following the principle mentioned of more distant objects in the same straight line seeming to move with the observer, when the position of the unerupted tooth altered to the right in the second film, we deduce it to be the more distant from the tube than the other teeth and, consequently, on the lingual side. (Figs. 196 and 197.)

Of course, the unerupted tooth might be one lying to the buccal side of the other teeth. In which case, it would appear on the second film farther to the left than it showed in the first film, indicating an apparent movement opposite in direction to that in which the tube was shifted, and thus harmonizing with the principle upon which the technique is based. (Figs. 198 and 199.)

This system, originated by Clark, was first outlined in Bennett's *Science and Practice of Dental Surgery,* and though of sound scientific and technical value, it was not esteemed or employed generally until Ivy recognized its high importance in his *Interpretations of Dental and Maxillary Roentgenograms.*

While Clark's theory is applicable in good practice to all cases where unerupted teeth are suspected or looked for, nevertheless, there is a greater assurance of better results where the region of the

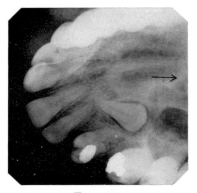

Fig. 198 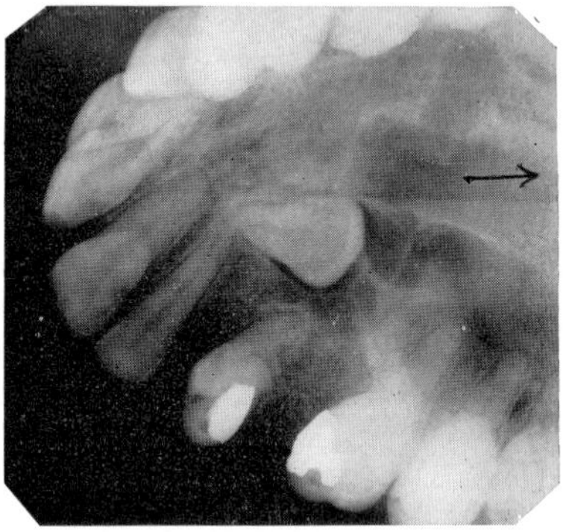   Fig. 199

Fig. 198.—Showing impacted canine to be localized in Fig. 199.

Fig. 199.—Tube was moved posteriorly as indicated by arrows; the canine has moved in the opposite direction to that of the movement of the tube; therefore, the canine lies on the buccal side.

mandibular third molar is involved by following the technique suggested by Dr. Fred Miller (1914), and later popularized by Winter.

Miller's technique for the localization of the mandibular third molar also requires the use of two films and the making of two exposures. Ordinary small intra-oral dental film is used.

For the first roentgenogram, the film is placed in the mouth parallel with the mean plane of the teeth; the anterior border of the film must not extend anteriorly farther than the mesial border of the first molar. The rays are directed perpendicularly to the mean tangent of the molars, thus securing the proper posterior dimensions of the molars and any indication of the displacement of the third molar.

For the second roentgenogram, the film is placed over the occlusal surfaces of the mandibular molars, the anterior border of the film extending no farther forward than the mesial border of the first molar. The posterior border of the film should extend over the retromolar triangle.

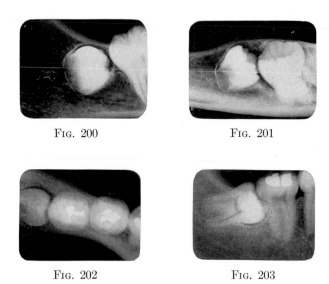

FIG. 200   FIG. 201

FIG. 202   FIG. 203

FIGS. 200 to 203.—Miller's technique for the localization of the mandibular third molar.

FIGS. 200 and 201.—Mandibular third molar in process of development. Fig. 200, lateral view, shows mesial inclination. Fig. 201, occlusal view, shows lingual inclination.

FIG. 202.—Occlusal view, shows impacted mandibular third molar in median lines without lateral displacement.

FIG. 203.—Lateral view, shows mesial inclination of impacted mandibular third molar and its relation to the second molar in the same plane.

The patient must be instructed to hold the film in position by a light bite; and while so held between the teeth, the head of the patient is tilted backward until the plane of occlusion is perpendicular to the floor, and the rays then directed perpendicularly to the plane of the film through the lower border of the mandible in the region of the third molar. The results should show any lateral displacement of the third molar. (Figs. 200 and 203.)

In addition to the superiority of the Miller technique for localizing impacted mandibular third molars, it may be suggested as also superior for localizing any other impacted mandibular teeth and for localizing foreign bodies, broken instruments, for example, that are found in the mandible from time to time. (Figs. 204 and 205.)

Root Fragments.—To localize root fragments in edentulous mouths there should be prepared a film-holder with an attached wire extending at right angles to the anterior border of the holder. At right angles to this wire, 20 mm. from the anterior border of the holder, a second wire is attached (Fig. 206) which shall be termed the "localizing wire."

Setting the film in the holder, with this localizing wire over the surface of the film (Fig. 207), the holder is inserted into the mouth, and a registration of the anterior border of the film-holder made on the tissues by marking with an indelible pencil. That done, the

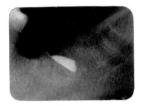 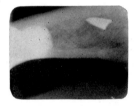

Fig. 204.—Lateral.   Fig. 205.—Occlusal.

Figs. 204 and 205.—Localizing broken instruments by the use of two roentgenograms—under Miller's technique.

exposure is made, the film developed and the distance of the root fragment from the anterior border measured. This residual root area is then marked upon the tissues at the same distance from the originally made indelible pencil line as it appears distant on the film, the localizing wire aiding thereby to obtain exactitude in localization by reason of its positive indication of distance and the possibility of gauging position in relation to it.

Thus the operator is permitted to make the incision for the removal of the root fragment with the least amount of tissue disturbance.

There is another means of localizing roots in edentulous mouths, one not requiring the film-holder. This comprises the use of a metal backing of any old film, so cut out to present a strip approximately $\frac{1}{8}$ inch in width, the length of the backing, with extensions at each end and in the center of approximately 5 mm., and fastened

to the emulsion side of the film packet to be used. Adhesive tape
or paper will answer the purpose of fasteners. (Fig. 208.)

After inserting packet in the mouth, a mark with an indelible
pencil is made at the anterior border of the film.

Exposure is made, and
care should be exercised to
retain this strip attachment,
for upon development of the

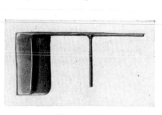
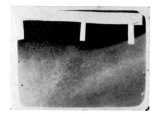

Fig. 206   Fig. 207

Fig. 206.—Small film-holder with localizing wire attached.

Fig. 207.—Film-holder with film in position, showing localizing wire in
position.

film we seen the outline of the strip and, in relation to any one or
two of the three extensions of the strip, the exact position of the
residual root.

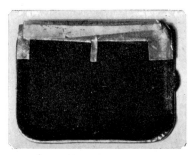

Fig. 208   Fig. 209

Fig. 208.—Strip of old film backing, cut and fastened on the emulsion
side of the film packet.

Fig. 209.—Illustrating the localization of a residual root in an edentulous mouth, the middle extension being over the root.

First noting the position of the affected area as shown on the
negative, the binding adhesive tape or paper is removed and the
strip replaced in the mouth in the identical position it occupied

during the exposure, as determined by the indelible mark on the tissues. Thus we may gauge the exact spot for the incision by the guide of the strip extensions and the distance from any one extension that the root appears in the film. (Fig. 209.) The film packet is placed in the edentulous mouth in the suspected area. A mark is

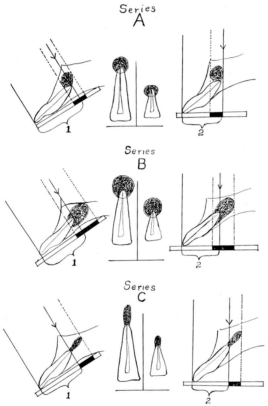

Fig. 210.—Topographical indications of periapical bone lesions. (Cieszynski.)

then made on the tissue with an indelible pencil at the anterior border of the film packet. The film is then exposed and developed. The distance from the anterior border of the film to the root fragment or foreign object is measured and this measurement transferred to the mouth, using the indelible mark on the tissue and measuring posteriorly. By this means we may accurately gauge the proper area for the incision.

TOPOGRAPHICAL INDICATIONS OF PERIAPICAL LESIONS.

"The topographical position of periapical bone cavities is ascertained by a constructive and comparative method." This is the statement of Cieszynski (1912), and by following his technique we may easily locate the position of the bony cavity. For this, two roentgenograms are taken: The first to give the normal length of the tooth; the second to show the tooth with shortened axis on the bite film. A reference to Fig. 210 will explain concisely the proper position of the film and the angle of the rays for these exposures.

Series A.—In the outline showing the tooth of normal length, the shadow of the bone cavity appears above the apex of the tooth, while in the foreshortened outline it appears below the apex of the tooth. And from the application of the theories governing shadow projections, we discover, therefore, that the diseased area is situated near the labial plate.

Series B.—The shadow appears both below and above the apex of the tooth in both outlines, and, therefore, the center of the disease lies near the region of the palate.

Series C.—In the outline showing normal length of the tooth, as well as in the foreshortened outline, a cavity is apparently above the apex and in the direction of the long axis of the tooth. In the outline showing normal length, the shadow has a longer and narrower appearance, while in the foreshortened outline it seems globular and diminished. In neither outline does the cavity area appear superimposed over any portion of the root. The disease area, therefore, lies directly over the apex of the tooth.

The foregoing illustrations (Fig. 210) incorporate the ideas originally enunciated by Cieszynski.

CHAPTER VI.

DENTAL ROENTGEN–RAY FILMS.

MANUFACTURERS of photographic plates and films have produced dental roentgen-ray films that conform to nearly every demand. The Eastman Kodak Company seems to be the leader in this field, and has made it possible for the roentgenologist to select a film which will assure him the proper contrasts. The various types of film from which you may select are as follows:

DENTAL ROENTGEN–RAY FILM FOR INTRA–ORAL WORK.

These films are in three speeds, designated "regular," "extra fast," and "radiatized." The "regular" and "extra fast" films are single coated, the emulsion being on only one side of the base, with a dull appearance on the emulsion side and a glossy appearance on the opposite, the non-emulsion, side. The best results are obtained with the regular film, as the emulsion has greater latitude for error, These films also have on the non-emulsion side a thin covering of gelatin to prevent curling.

The radiatized film has an emulsion on both sides of the base. It is obtained in one speed only. The identification of this film is made possible by observing the small dot on the film, the concaved side of the dot correspond-to the non-emulsion side of the regular film.

When these films are mounted in the film-holders for interpretation, the non-emulsion side should face the operator. This serves a two-fold purpose: it protects the emulsion and it standardizes the routine of mounting so that the films are viewed as though the operator were looking outward from the inside of the mouth. The right side of the mouth will show on the right side of the mount. (Fig. 212.)

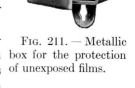

FIG. 211. — Metallic box for the protection of unexposed films.

There are various films on the market having special type packets. Besides those already mentioned, the most popular are the Bolin film, supplied with a rubber covering and of value in extremely sore mouths, and the Buck X-Ograph film, which has a stiff metallic back, and is supplied in three speeds—"slow or regular," "blue base or intermediate," and "fast."

The Occlusal Film.—The occlusal film (Eastman occlusal film) is of great importance, enabling the operator to obtain a general view of the palate or the floor of the mouth. It derives its name, bite film, from the position in which it is held in the mouth, that being horizontal and parallel with the plane of occlusion. It is of the slow or regular emulsion.

Inter-proximal Bite-wing Film.—The bite-wing film in inter-proximal examinations discloses more accurately signs of caries in the crowns of teeth, atrophic changes in the alveolar septa, and constructive and destructive changes in the pulp.

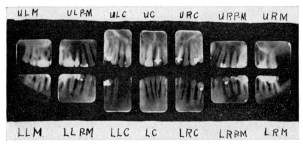

Fig. 212.—Method of mounting and type of mount used for a fourteen film exposure of the mouth.

Its function is most important in revealing caries at inception as well as recurrent under fillings, both of which the clinical examinations often miss.

If we would preserve the teeth in the state of health with which Nature endowed us, this type of examination should be used periodically from childhood.

DENTAL ROENTGEN-RAY FILMS FOR EXTRA-ORAL WORK.

In this type of film the emulsion is coated on both sides of the transparent base. Increased speed is obtained thereby. They may be used for direct exposures of all classes and should be loaded either in cassettes or special roentgen-ray exposure-holders (Eastman). They are best used with intensifying screens, and must surely be marked carefully at the time of exposure, because of the necessity of later identification of the side to which they had been applied.

The Intensifying Screen (Fig. 214).—When roentgen-rays strike the emulsion of a film, less than 1 per cent of their energy is absorbed, the remaining 99 per cent passing through without performing any useful work. It is the absorption that governs the formation of the latent image. Therefore, any method devised to utilize part of this 99 per cent waste means a decidedly advantageous attainment.

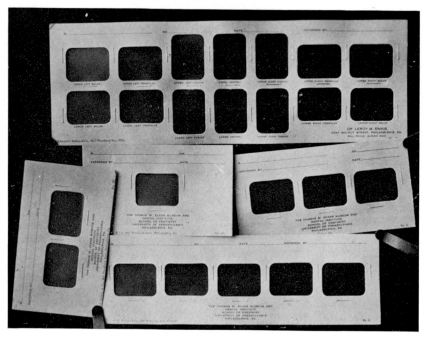

Fig. 213.—Various types of film mounts.

It is known that certain chemicals have the property of absorbing roentgen-rays and emitting their energy as ordinary light. This property is called "fluorescence." Calcium tungstate, a white crystalline salt, has this property. When finely powdered, mixed with a suitable binder and coated in a thin, smooth layer on a light flexible support, it is known as an intensifying screen. When its use is indicated the duplitized film is placed between two intensifying screens, which results in the absorbing of the wasted roentgen-rays and the returning of the emitted ordinary light back to the emulsion to intensify the photographic result. The function of the intensifying screen is to reduce the time of exposure, thereby obtaining a better result.

Cassettes (Fig. 215).—In acutal use, intensifying screens are mounted in pairs in rigid holders called cassettes in order that perfect contact may be obtained between emulsion and the screens.

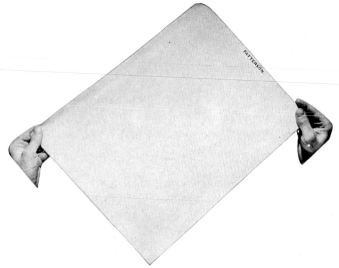

Fig. 214.—Patterson intensifying screen.

The duplitized film is placed in the cassette, so that the emulsion is in direct contact with the screens. All paper covering must be

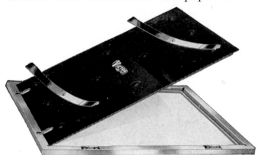

Fig. 215.—Victor cassette.

removed from the film and particular care taken to prevent any dust or chemicals coming in contact with the screens, as such foreign substances absorb the light and cause a spot to be formed on the film when developed.

Static.—Removal of the film from the cassette should be made with care. It should be lifted gently, never drawn across the surface of the intensifying screen. Especially so is this important when there is the least humidity in the atmosphere; for the least friction between the film and the screen will surely discharge static electricity that may cause the film to be exposed, resulting as in Fig. 216.

The Identification of Roentgenograms.—Intra-oral roentgenograms may be readily distinguished as to whether they are right or left

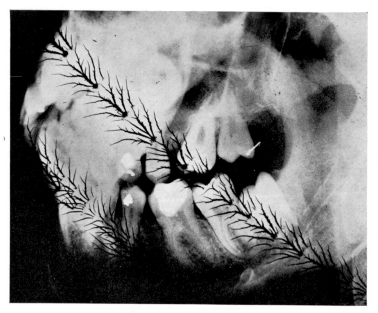

Fig. 216.—Showing radiolucent streaks across the film caused by the film being exposed to static electricity while being removed improperly from the cassette.

by proper observation: Viewing the film with the shiny side toward the observer gives the lingual aspect, the observer visualizing himself sitting inside the patient's mouth and looking out, and whatever is to the observer right is to the patient's right.

For example, in viewing the maxillary molar teeth, with the apices pointing up and the shiny side of the film toward the observer, if the distal of this region (which in this case is the third molar) appears to the right, then it is the maxillary right molar region. If the distal appears to the left, then it is the maxillary left molar region.

THE CHEMISTRY OF PHOTOGRAPHIC MATERIALS.

The art of photography is founded upon the fact that the compounds of silver, and especially its compounds with chlorine, bromine and iodine, are sensitive to light.

Sensitive photographic materials consist of paper, film or glass, coated with a sensitive layer which holds in suspension silver bromide or silver chloride. This sensitive layer is called the emulsion.

A photographic emulsion consists then of the silver salts suspended in a solution of gelatin. In preparing the materials the gelatin is soaked in water until it is swollen and then dissolved in warm water. The necessary potassium bromide or sodium chloride is thereupon added to the solution until all is dissolved. Silver nitrate in sufficient quantity to react with the amount of salts used is dissolved in water, this solution, added slowly to the solution of gelatin and salt, producing a precipitate of the silver compound. The mixing is all done in the dark-room. Without the silver nitrate, the silver compound would settle to the bottom and no emulsion would form. The function of the gelatin is to prevent the settling and keep the silver compound suspended and the evenly precipitated silver salt distributed through the solution. This emulsion is then coated on some support like paper, film or glass, and cooled. The gelatin sets, and when dried we get a smooth coating of dry gelatin containing the sensitive silver compound.

Negative-making materials, such as plates and films, always contain silver bromide with a small addition of silver iodide. The different degrees of sensitiveness are obtained by the temperature and duration of the heat which the emulsions undergo during manufacture, the most sensitive emulsions, the faster emulsions, being heated to higher temperatures and for a longer time than are the slower emulsions.

The most important chemicals contributing to make a photographic emulsion are:

Silver nitrate, obtained by dissolving metallic silver in nitric acid. The silver replaces the hydrogen of the acid and forms silver nitrate, which is crystallized out of the solution and obtained in colorless, transparent plates.

Potassium chloride is a white salt, similar to sodium chloride.

Potassium bromide occurs as a colorless cubical crystal and is generally pure, and soluble in water.

Silver bromide is obtained by the addition of a solution of silver nitrate to a solution of potassium bromide. The reaction occurs as follows:

$$AgNo_2 + KBr = AgBr + KNO_3$$
Silver nitrate.   Potassium bromide.   Silver bromide.   Potassium nitrate.

The gelatin entering into the manufacture of photographic emulsions is obtained from the bones and skins of animals, and has curious and valuable properties. It belongs to a class of substances known as colloids, a derivation from a Greek word, meaning "gummy." It will not dissolve in cold water, but swells, and absorbs the water. If the water is heated the gelatin will dissolve.

When the gelatin dries, it shrinks, and this characteristic of swelling when wet and shrinking when dry is of great importance in photography. As warm water will dissolve gelatin, it is imperative to observe carefully the temperature of solutions in which the emulsion will be placed.

THE CHEMISTRY OF DEVELOPMENT.

When a photographic emulsion is exposed for a short time to light, the change that takes place is so minute it cannot be detected by ordinary means, but once the exposed material is placed in a chemical solution (the "developer"), the chlorine or bromine is taken away from the silver, and the black metallic silver which remains behind forms the image. The photographic emulsion acts as a storehouse for light energy, the emulsion retaining its original appearance until it is placed in suitable developing solutions.

The final image consists or is made up of microscopic grains of black metallic silver; for the microscopic crystalline grains of the sensitive silver salt in the original emulsion (the bromide) disappear in the developer, the crystals break up, and a tiny coke-like mass of metallic silver remains behind in exactly the same position as the bromide crystals from which they were formed.

The removal of the bromide from the metallic silver is known chemically as "reduction." (This chemical reduction must not be confused with the photographic operation known as the reducing of a negative, which is the weakening of an over-dense negative; the term there refers simply to the removal of the silver and is not used in the chemical sense.)

Chemical reducers have an affinity for oxygen, and must liberate the metals from their salts; so developing solutions must contain chemical reducers. Reducing agents used in the developer must be able to reduce the exposed silver bromide, but without affecting

12

unexposed silver bromide, so that their affinity must be within certain narrow bounds. Developing agents are limited to a very few substances, almost all of which are chemically derived from benzene, a coal-tar distillate.

Two chemicals used in the developing solution which are reducing agents, and have a definite action on a photographic emulsion, are:

1. Hydroquinone, made from benzene, and much better for our use than any other agent because, when used in conjunction with elon, it produces a developer which will keep for a long period of time.

2. Elon, monomethyl paramidophenol sulphate, a by-product of the manufacture of dyes, treated with methyl alcohol.

These agents have different actions during the period of development. They must be used conjointly to attain successful results. Images developed with hydroquinone come up very slowly but gain density steadily. Hydroquinone is affected very readily by the slightest change in temperature, or by the addition of a small amount of sodium or potassium bromide, while elon, when used alone in the developer, brings the image up very quickly all over the plate, gains density slowly, is not affected by a slight change of temperature, and is not affected to any great degree by sodium or potassium bromide. These differences in the developing agents depend upon the chemical nature of the substances themselves, and constitute what is called the "reduction potential" of the developer. A high reduction potential enables a developer to continue to develop more nearly at a normal rate under such adverse circumstances as low temperature or the presence of bromide. So from the action of the agents we can determine their potential.

Measuring the developing agents this way, hydroquinone has a very low potential. Elon will make the image flash up all over at once, and start development very quickly, producing detail. Hydroquinone, slower in action, brings up the high lights of the image first, the shadows not appearing until the high lights are somewhat developed, thereby giving contrast. Therefore, if both detail and contrast be desired, it is essential to use agents of both high and low potentials.

These agents cannot develop at all when used by themselves, and in order to do their work must be in an alkali solution, the energy depending upon the amount of alkali present. As alkalis govern the energy of the developer, it is highly important that only the proper amount be used. Too little alkali will slow up the action of the developer. Too much alkali will tend to produce a chemical fog. And as alkalis also soften the gelatin of the emulsion, too much alkali will produce over-swelling, causing frilling or blisters in warm weather.

Two kinds of alkalis are used in development: the caustic and the carbonized.

Caustic alkalis are used very little in our ordinary developing. But the so-called "minute" developer sometimes used is caustic, and great care must be taken when working with this solution as the caustic alkali used, caustic soda (NaOH) is injurious to the skin. In developing, the alkalis generally used are the carbonates—the salts of carbonic acid (N_2CO_3). Sodium carbonate is one. It is used in the form which contains 98 per cent carbonate and a small amount of residual water, and accelerates development by opening the pores of the emulsion. It is obtained by heating sodium bicarbonate.

$$\underset{\text{Sodium bicarbonate.}}{2NaHCO_3} \quad + \quad Heat \quad = \quad \underset{\text{Sodium carbonate.}}{Na_2CO_3} \quad + \quad \underset{\text{Carbon dioxide.}}{CO_2} \quad + \quad \underset{\text{Water.}}{H_2O}$$

Developers have a great affinity for oxygen, and because of the oxygen in the air, solutions containing only the developing agent and alkali would be spoiled rapidly by the process of oxidation from the air. By adding to the developing solution sulphite of soda, which has a strong affinity for oxygen and is easily oxidized into sulphate of soda, the developer is thereby protected from the oxygen, and its life prolonged.

Sodium sulphite is prepared by blowing sulphur dioxide gas into a solution of carbonate of soda. And as the sulphite readily oxidizes and forms a sulphate, which is not a preservative, care must be taken not to use any sulphite which has effloresced to any extent. The desiccated salt containing about 95 per cent of pure sulphite is the salt used in developing.

If we use a solution with a reducer, a preservative and an alkali, the developing process would probably be too rapid. Therefore, it is necessary in our solution to have potassium bromide. Occurring as colorless crystals, cubical in shape and generally pure, it functions as a restrainer, preventing both too rapid developing and fogging of the transparent areas. Summarizing the foregoing, a developing solution should be composed of the following formulæ:

Hydroquinone—oxidizing agent, giving contrast	128	grains
Elon—oxidizing agent, giving detail	32	"
Sodium sulphite, preservative	$1\frac{3}{5}$	ounces
Sodium carbonate, alkali	$1\frac{3}{5}$	"
Potassium bromide, restrainer	12	grains
Water (distilled), vehicle	32	ounces

Distilled water should be the vehicle in all developing solutions. Other waters may contain chemicals which will go into chemical combination with the chemicals of the developing solution and have a deleterious effect on the silver bromide salts of the emulsion.

THE CHEMISTRY OF FIXATION.

After development the undeveloped silver bromide salts are removed by immersion of the negative or print in what is called the "fixing" bath. Only a few substances will dissolve silver bromide, and one universally used in modern photography is sodium thiosulphate ($Na_2S_2O_3$), known as hyposulphite of soda, or more commonly as hypo.

Thiosulphate of soda can be made by boiling together sodium sulphite and sulphur, the sulphur combining with the sodium sulphite according to the equation:

$$Na_2SO_3 \quad + \quad S \quad = \quad Na_2S_2O_3$$

Sodium sulphite.   Sulphur.   Hypo.

In the process of fixation the silver bromide is dissolved in the hypo by combining with it to form a compound sodium thiosulphate. There exist two of these compounds (thiosulphates), one being almost insoluble in water, the other being very soluble. As long as the fixing-bath has any appreciable fixing-power, the soluble compound only is formed.

Fixing is accomplished by means of hypo only, but materials are usually transferred from the developer to the fixing-bath with very little rinsing, so that a good deal of developer is carried over into the fixing-bath, turning it brown, and staining negatives or prints. To avoid this, the bath has sulphite of soda added to it as a preservative against oxidation, and the preservative action is greater, of course, if the bath is kept in a slightly acid state. In order to prevent the gelatin from swelling and softening, it is also usual to add some hardening agent to the fixing-bath, so that instead of containing only hypo, a fixing-bath will contain in addition sulphite, an acid and a hardener.

The developer drippings carried over into the fixing-bath are, however, alkaline; and consequently in a fixing-bath which is used for any length of time a considerable amount of acid is required, since a small amount would soon be completely neutralized by the developer carried over. Thus arises the difficulty in requiring a large amount of acid present, and yet protecting the fixing-bath against being strongly acid. The protection against the difficulty lies in certain acids that are very weak in acidity and yet can neutralize alkali successfully. Large amounts of these acids can be added without making the bath of such acidity as to precipitate the sulphur.

The strongest acids are the mineral acids, such as sulphuric and hydrochloric, while the weakest are the organic acids, those made from vegetable products, such as citric and acetic. As we require a large amount of a weak acid, the best for our purpose is acetic acid.

Acetic acid in its diluted form is a vinegar resulting from the fermentation of alcohol, the stronger acid being made by neutralizing with lime the crude acetic acid prepared by the destructive distillation of wood.

The commonest hardening agent is potash alum. The alums have the property of shrinking and tanning gelatin. Chrome alum, often used in the place of ordinary alum, has greater hardening power, its only disadvantage being its greenish color which makes the fixing-bath somewhat dark.

Chrome alum is a compound sulphate of potassium sulphate or ammonium sulphate with chromium sulphate occurring in violet crystals soluble in water.

It is very important not to over-work a fixing-bath. As it becomes saturated with silver, the film will carry this silver into the wash-water with it; and if the film is not properly washed the silver salt will adhere to the finised photograph and in time will decompose into silver sulphide, causing a yellowish stain.

Summarizing the foregoing, a fixing-solution should be composed of the chemical agents making up the following formulæ:

Water (distilled), vehicle	80 ounces
Hypo, silver bromide solvent	2 pounds

When dissolved add

Water (distilled), vehicle	10 ounces
Sodium bisulphite, preservative	3 "
Chrome alum, hardener	100 grains

Make up to gallon by the addition of distilled water

or

Water, vehicle	64 ounces
Hypo, silver bromide solvent	16 "

When dissolved add

Alum (powdered), hardener	1 ounce
Acetic acid, 28 per cent, acidifier	3 ounces
Sodium sulphite, preservative	1 ounce
Water, vehicle	8 ounces

THE CHEMISTRY OF REDUCTION.

By reduction in photography is meant the removal of some silver from the image so as to produce a less intense image. Thus, in case of an over-developed film or an over-exposed film, there will be an excess of density and contrast, and this requires the removal of the excess density.

All film reducers being oxidizing agents, they will act as a photographic reducer, and will remove silver, but various oxidizing agents behave differently in respect to the high lights and shadows of the image. Reducing solutions can be divided in three clases:

1. Cutting reducers.
2. True scale reducers.
3. Flattening reducers.

With need limited to the film, the cutting reducers are the ones important to understand. Cutting reducers remove an equal amount of silver from all parts of the image and consequently remove a larger proportion of the image from the shadows than from the high lights of the negative.

The typical cutting reducer is known as Farmer's reducer, consisting of enough *potassium ferricyanide* solution, added to plain hypo solution (not acid fixing-bath), 1 to 4, to make lemon-yellow color. After reducing in this solution the film must be washed thoroughly.

Or a satisfactory cutting reducer may be very easily made as follows:

Solution A

Potassium ferricyanide	1 ounce
Water (distilled)	16 ounces

Solution B

Hypo (crystals)	1 ounce
Water (distilled)	16 ounces

Keep in brown bottles and use equal parts of A and B. The film may be reduced immediately after it has been fixed. Immerse in reducing solution for one or two seconds, place in water, examine film for correct density, and place in water to wash. If upon the examination the density desired has not been secured, repeat operation until proper density is obtained. The reducer must be used immediately, for it decomposes rapidly when mixed.

The potassium ferricyanide oxidizes the silver in the film emulsion to silver ferrocyanide and the hypo dissolves the silver ferrocyanide.

THE CHEMISTRY OF WASHING.

Laws governing washing are distinctly chemical in nature, and the importance of washing in photography justifies greater attention than is usually paid to the subject.

The object in washing negatives or prints is to remove from them the chemicals of the fixing-bath. In the first place, it should not be necessary to wash out silver compounds, but only the chemicals of the fixing-bath. If an over-worked fixing-bath is used, silver compounds will be present during washing, and must be very completely removed, so that if work has to be hurried and the time of washing must be cut down it is most important that fixing should be complete.

In fixation silver bromide is dissolved by the hypo, and forms two compounds of silver thiosulphates, one almost insoluble in water, the other very soluble. As long as the fixing-bath has any appreciable fixing-power the soluble compound only is formed. This first insoluble compound is invisible, and if a negative is transferred to the washing tank as soon as it is visibly clear, some of the insoluble silver hypo compound will still remain in the negative when it is dry. Therefore, the hypo should be kept fresh at all times, and the film allowed to remain in the solution for some time after it has cleared. This will simplify the washing.

It is a common belief that plates can be washed more rapidly in warm water than in cold. This is a mistake. Diffusion must take place in gelatin, and the warmer the water the more the gelatin swells, and its swelling hinders the diffusion in about the same proportion as the rise in temperature accelerates it; so that a wash should be about the general ordinary temperature.

The actual time of washing may be understood by remembering that the amount of hypo remaining in the gelatin is continually halved in the same period of time as the washing proceeds. An average negative will give up one-half its hypo in two minutes; so that at the end of two minutes a half of the hypo will be remaining in it; after four minutes, one-quarter; after six minutes, one-eighth; and so on. In a very short time the amount of hypo remaining would be little. This, however, assumes that the negative is continually exposed to fresh water; for negatives should be subjected to a continuous stream of fresh water. If this is not possible, the water should be changed often in the wash-tray.

TEMPERATURE.

Most chemical reactions proceed more rapidly as the temperature is increased, and this is true of all the reactions involved in photography. Developers and fixers act much more rapidly when warm than when cold.

Different reducers do not react the same at a given temperature; for example: At low temperature hydroquinone is very inert, while elon is not decreased in its rate of action to the same extent. At high temperatues the hydroquinone is increased in its activity far more than elon. So in using a mixed hydroquinone and elon

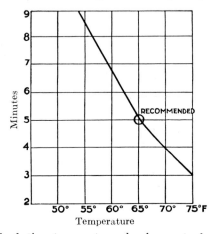

Fig. 217.—Standard time-temperature development chart for Eastman Dupli-Tized X-Ray and Dental Films.

After carefully taking temperature of developer, trace a vertical line on the chart from the temperature line until it intersects the curve, then trace a horizontal line from this point to the left margin. This will indicate the correct time of development for Eastman Dupli-Tized X-Ray and Dental Films. (Eastman Kodak Company Medical Division, Rochester, New York.)

solution it is necessary to develop at a temperature of 65° F., at which the best results are obtained. (Fig. 217.)

DEVELOPMENT.

There are three methods of developing a photographic plate: The factoral method, the tray or visual method, and the tank method. But before discussing the various methods of developing, the dark-room should be considered. The dark-room should be so constructed that all outside sources of light may be excluded. It should be equipped with a red light—not simply a red-stained electric bulb, but one which affords ample light plus real safety, such as the Kodak safelight lamp. Red light is used because the red rays are chemically inactive. There should also be in the dark-room two glass graduates, one for mixing the developer and the other for mixing the hypo; and they should be so marked so as to prevent contamination of the hypo with the developer. Other necessities are trays and tanks for the various solutions, glass mix-

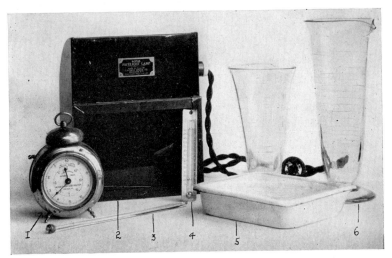

Fig. 218.—Essential equipment for the dark-room: 1, interval timer; 2, proper safelight lamp; 3, glass mixing-rod; 4, thermometer; 5, porcelain trays; 6, glass graduates.

ing-rods to stir the chemicals into solution, an interval timing-clock, and, most important of all, a thermometer. (Fig. 218.)

The chemicals for developing and fixing may be obtained from the manufacturer in their proper proportions and ready to mix in distilled water. They come in sizes which will make 1 gallon of solution or in sizes which will make 12 ounces of solution. It is advisable to obtain chemicals in this manner, because they are easily and quickly handled, and always fresh. They are put up in moisture-proof containers, as seen in Fig. 219. However, if one wishes to alter the formulæ or should desire for any reason to mix the chemicals, they may be obtained in bulk. (Fig. 220.)

It is very important to have proper containers for solutions. One very important guide in the selection of the containers is the amount of work to be done, for that factor controls the amount of

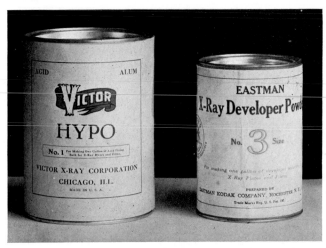

FIG. 219.—Hypo containing chrome alum. Developing powders. Gallon size.

solution used. However, for the average dental office, the Eastman dental 12-ounce film tank will answer all necessary purposes.

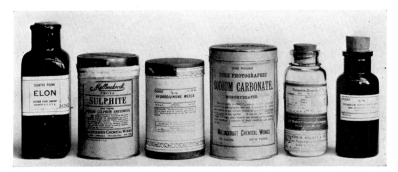

FIG. 220.—Chemicals used in developing, when desiring to change the formula from the standard.

Figs. 221, 222 and 223 illustrate the method in which they may be used. A porcelain tray, 10 by 12 inches in size, is filled with water; three small 12-ounce tanks, each labelled for their proper solutions, are placed in the tray of water. The purpose of the water is to keep the solutions at the proper temperature at all times; so in winter, when the solutions may be too cold, warm water

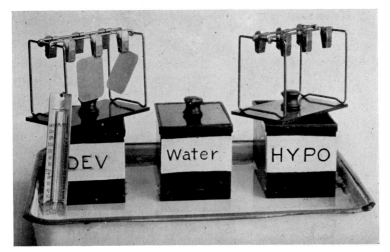

FIG. 221.—Eastman 12-ounce developing tanks with film-holders. Tanks are marked and placed in a tray containing water. They may be covered when not in use. The temperature of the solution may be maintained at 65° by adding either warm or cold water to the water surrounding the tanks.

may be placed in the tray until the solutions arrive at their proper temperature (65° F.); and just the reverse takes place in summer

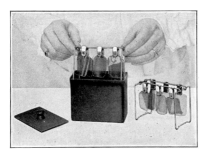

FIG. 222.—Eastman 12-ounce developing tank.

by adding cold water or ice to bring the solution down to the correct temperature. Water is never added to the developing solution or the hypo, for such dilution renders the solutions less active. This cardinal idea should be kept in mind at all times: the best results are obtained when the solutions are active and at the correct temperature.

These small tanks are of hard rubber and equipped with a lid made of the same material that protects the solutions when not in use from undergoing rapid oxidation from exposure to the air. The film hangers supplied for these tanks hold six films and are made of a metal which is not affected by the chemicals of the solution. (Fig. 222.) Of course, larger containers for the use of more solution

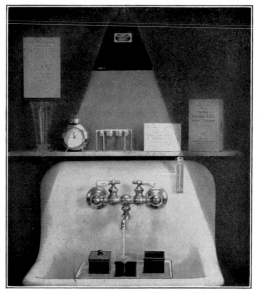

Fig. 223.—Well-equipped dark-room for the small amount of work done in the average dental office.

may be obtained from the various manufacturers. The one illustrated in Fig. 227 answers all general purposes, as it is practically a dark-room in itself. It should be particularly noted that the chief factor in keeping solutions for any length of time is the prevention of oxidation; so the covering should never be neglected. If the containers are not supplied with covers, one can easily be made with a piece of cork $\frac{1}{4}$ inch thick, cut to the size of the top of the container, *and covered with paraffine to prevent the solutions from coming in contact with the cork*. Cork will float on the solutions and prevent them from coming in contact with the air. (Fig. 224.)

Properly equipped, we may proceed with the developing process, and first consider the *factoral* method of developing. It is based on the knowledge that the total time of development of a plate bears a fixed relation to the time of appearance of the image. Therefore, the exposed film is placed in the developing solution (65° F.), the time is take from the moment the film is placed in the solution until the first sign of a reaction takes place, and this time is multiplied by the factor of the developer, which, for our developer, is 30. The result is then divided by 60, the number of seconds in one minute, and the result denotes the time the film should remain in the solution to be properly developed. For example: Take three films exposed under identical conditions except for time of exposure, one having had two seconds of exposure, another having had five seconds, and the third having had eight seconds' exposure. Upon developing, we find that the image on the two seconds'

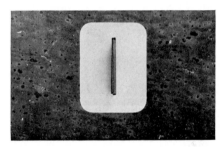

Fig. 224.—Cork cut to the size of the developing tank and which is allowed to float on the developer to protect it from the air. Note.—The cork should be coated with paraffine to prevent the solutions from penetrating into the cork.

exposure appears in fifteen seconds, the one on the five seconds' exposure appears in ten seconds, and the one on the eight seconds' exposure appears in five seconds. To find the precise time of proper development is now a mathematical procedure.

	Image time.		Factors.				Seconds		Developing period.
No. 1.	15 seconds	×	30	=	450	÷	60	=	$7\frac{1}{2}$ minutes
No 2.	10 seconds	×	30	=	300	÷	60	=	5 minutes
No 3.	5 seconds	×	30	=	150	÷	60	=	$2\frac{1}{2}$ minutes

By this method we have three films which are almost identical, have eliminated chance and established uniformity. But the majority of the developing is done by the *tray* or *visual* method, which may be assumed to be the most popular system.

The old method of placing a film in a developer and guessing when the film was properly developed has been superseded by a definitely established technique. From experience we know that a film properly exposed and placed in a fresh developer at 65° F. will be properly developed in five minutes. (Fig. 217.)

So now, when an exposure is made, the film is placed in the developing solution, our interval timing-clock is set for five minutes, and we proceed meanwhile with some other work. At the end of the five minutes the alarm sounds to remind us that development is complete. The film is then fixed; if it had been properly exposed it

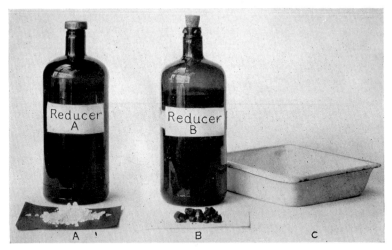

Fig. 225.—Chemicals used as reducing agents for over-developed films: A, hypo (crystals); B, potassium ferricyanide; C, special tray used for reducing only.

will be correctly developed. If, however, the film is too thin, we know that we have under-exposed the film, or if the film is too dense we know that we have over-exposed our film. Thus this simple method of developing not only eliminates procedures which seem difficult, but at the same time supplies a means or method of checking up on our exposures. If the tray method is followed as described, the operator will obtain satisfactory and uniform results.

The tank method of developing appeals to many of the foremost workers in the field as the more nearly ideal way than are any of the other systems. It is based on the action of a developer of a given strength, for a given length of time, at a given temperature. The great advantage of this method is uniform development. But like many ideals, it seems to be shunned and practically discarded. However, we seen in Fig. 226 a very useful tank for the purpose of

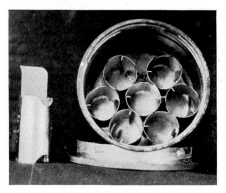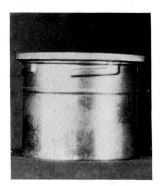

FIG. 226.—Tank for the development of small dental films.

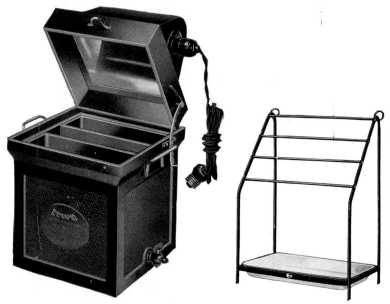

FIG. 227.—The Mabee tank with safelight in cover.

FIG. 228.—Victor film drying rack.

developing dental films by this method. The small tubes cannot be employed if one uses radiatized film, the film which has the emulsion on both sides; for the emulsion would come in contact with the metal when wet and would adhere, and the film would be spoiled by reason of the emulsion being torn.

It can easily be understood that if an under-exposed film is developed for five minutes it will be very thin, and should be discarded. Intensification has been suggested for such film. But this operation does not give satisfactory results. On the other hand, if an over-exposed film is developed for five minutes, and the result

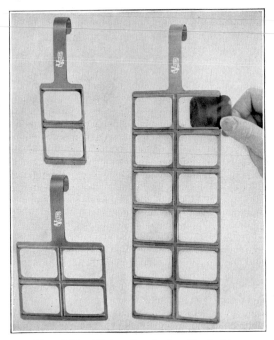

Fig. 229.—Victor developing film-holders.

shows very dense, this density may be remedied by the process of reduction in bringing the film back to its proper density by the removal of the excess metallic silver. Reduction can be carried out immediately after taking the film from the fixing-solution. Reducing-solution should be ready for use at all times, and should be kept in brown bottles to protect against the light. (Fig. 225.) The operator must remember the importance of washing the film. It should always be washed between solutions, and, after it has been fixed, should remain in running water for at least twenty minutes before drying.

Metol Dermatitis.—Metol dermatitis, often mentioned as metol poisoning, is caused more by the alkalies in the developing solution then by the metol.

Symptoms.—Hands become cracked, gashed, papulated.

Treatment.—Keep hands immersed for two hours daily in a basin of water continuously kept very hot until condition disappears. Care should be used in handling developing solutions by those at all susceptible. The hands should be most thoroughly washed in very hot water after being in contact with the solution, and, in addition, a good grease ointment or skin lotion should be rubbed well into the hands after such a washing. This will tend to keep the skin from cracking.

PRACTICAL HINTS FOR THE DARK-ROOM.

All necessary equipment should have a definite place in the dark-room, for once the lights are out and developing begun, it may be found necessary to use some piece of equipment not already in use. If it has a proper place it may be easily reached; otherwise something may be broken while groping for it in the dark. Clean towels should always be in the dark-room, and the hands should be dry when handling films, otherwise the films when finished will contain finger marks which cannot be removed.

Great care should be taken not to allow the emulsion side of the film to come in contact with the side or bottom of the developing tank, as the emulsion will adhere to the tank and will not develop at the contact point; for when the film is placed in the fixing-bath the silver bromide salts which have not been reduced will be dissolved, leaving a clear emulsion having the appearance of a radiopaque area as seen in Figs. 230 and 231. Radiopaque streaks may also appear on the films when they over-lap each other in the developing tank. Re-used clips that have not been thoroughly washed after they have been once immersed in hypo will also cause streaks; for, when in contact with the developer, the dried hypo dissolves and runs down over the emulsion of the film, dissolving the silver bomide before it is developed.

The same care should be taken when films are in the fixing-bath. If the emulsion comes in contact with the sides of the tank the hypo does not have the opportunity of removing the unused silver bromide salts where the emulsion is in contact. Therefore, when the film is removed it will contain areas which are dark, having the appearance of a radiolucent area. (Fig. 233.)

13

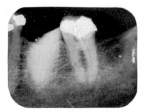 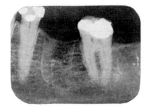

Fig. 230   Fig. 231

Figs. 230 and 231.—Fig. 230, film allowed to rest against tank during development, showing radiopaque area in the region of the mandibular first molar. Fig. 231, roentgenogram of the same area, showing no pathological condition present, the radiopaque area not appearing because the film was properly developed.

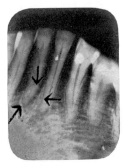 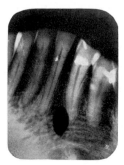

Fig. 232   Fig. 233

Figs. 232 and 233.—Fig. 232, film with water spot; a drop of water having come in contact with the emulsion after it had dried. Fig. 233, duplicate of Fig. 232, except the emulsion was in contact with the side of the tank in the fixing-bath preventing the removal of the unused salts, thus making it possibly appear as if some abnormal condition existed in the apical region of the mandibular canine, which Fig. 232 refutes.

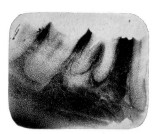 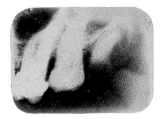

Fig. 234   Fig. 235

Figs. 234 and 235.—Films washed in water, which was too warm, and showing a pitted appearance (reticulation).

The temperature of the water in which the films are washed is of great importance. If the temperature is too high, the films will become pitted or reticulated. (Figs. 234 and 235.) This is caused by the softening of the gelatin of the emulsion. It may be prevented by using a hardener in the fixing-bath, which hardens the emulsion, and, additionally, by keeping the wash-water below 80° F.

Care should also be taken in not allowing drops of water to come in contact with the emulsion after it has dried, otherwise the film will be spotted. (Fig. 232.)

If, however, drops of water should come in contact with the dry emulsion, the entire film should immediately be immersed in water for five minutes, which will allow the entire emulsion to expand, after which the film is allowed to dry with no water-mark evident.

CHAPTER VII.

ROUTINE EXAMINATION OF THE ORAL CAVITY.

INTERPRETATION of roentgenograms is not a demonstration of expert crystal-gazing. While it is true that some pathological conditions are unmistakably revealed by the roentgenogram, there are many which can be diagnosed intelligently only by a thorough consideration of both the case history and the roentgenogram.

The person upon whom the interpretation of the roentgenograms devolves, therefore, should know as much as possible of the history of the teeth of the patient, swellings, pain, or any condition of troublesome nature, as well as any previous treatment.

A general survey of the mouth and associated structures must be made. It is the only way for the examiner to obtain a clue as to the nature and extent of the roentgenographic examination required. The presence of suppurating sinuses, swellings and other symptoms may then be more surely defined.

The next important step is the determination of the vitality of the teeth. For this, a roentgenographic examination is made and the doubtful teeth noted; and any doubtful teeth may then be tested for their vitality by one of two methods—the electric test or the thermal test.

To attempt any roentgenographic interpretation without having all possible knowledge of existing conditions surrounding the involved area, and particularly as to the vitality of the pulp, may lead to inaccurate diagnoses and erroneous advice, with dire consequential results following.

The Electric Vitality Test.—The electric vitality test has proved the most satisfactory, as well as the simplest, system to answer the necessities of most cases.

The oldest electric method for testing tooth vitality, and today the least used, is by means of the Faradic battery. (Fig. 236.)

The Faradic apparatus consists of a $1\frac{1}{2}$ volt dry-cell battery, an interrupter, a coil and two electrodes; the current passing from the dry cell through an interrupter and thence to a coil, by means of which the current is changed to one of high voltage and low amperage. In making tests, the negative electrode is placed in the hand of the patient. The point of the positive electrode is wrapped with a wisp of cotton moistened with water, and, after the tooth under

(196)

examination is dried, the moistened electrode is placed on the surface of the enamel of the tooth. The current is thereupon turned on and increased or decreased by passing the primary current in or out of the secondary. At no time is it possible for the patient to receive any current greater than that supplied by the dry-cell battery used. Those who use a Faradic battery device for vitality testing, or any device where a hand electrode is employed, should acquaint themselves with the fact that the point at which the patient reports feeling the current will vary as the contact and

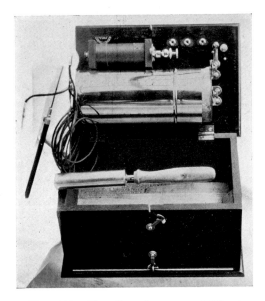

Fig. 236.—Faradic pulp-tester. (Pilling.)

moisture employed varies. For instance, if a patient grasps the hand electrode lightly, holding the same with the tips of two or three fingers, far more electric current will be required to obtain a response than if the patient grasped the electrode tightly in the palm of the hand and held the electrode firmly. If the hand is dry more current is required, while if the hand is moist, due to perspiration, the electric current will meet far less resistance and the response is obtained from the patient with less current.

Because of these variables the findings obtained by this method vary greatly. It is, therefore, advisable to employ means which allow the operator to control the variables to a greater extent.

The Burton Vitalometer.—This is a modern, widely used apparatus which produces a Faradic current. The vitalometer operates from the 100- to 120-volt line current (alternating) which has passed through a special current controller known as a power governor. The power governor is placed in the regular commercial current outlet and a cord connects the power governor to the vitalometer. The vitalometer cannot be operated without the power governor, since the power governor allows only a very low voltage and a very low amperage to pass into the vitalometer. (Fig. 237.)

The current which passes into the vitalometer is "stepped up" by the use of a primary and secondary induction coil, and before the current passes out of the vitalometer into the electrode it passes through an automatic interrupter. This makes the current which enters the tooth a highly pulsating Faradic current. The voltage is regulated by a slide adjuster from nothing to 2000 volts of electromotive force. The actual amount of amperage used is very little, averaging about $\frac{1}{10}$ milliampère.

The electrodes are so constructed that both positive and negative terminals are placed in contact with the tooth being tested. This eliminates the need for hand or cheek electrodes. This also eliminates body or hand resistance as a factor in testing vitality. Since the current is directed directly into the tooth, we assume that no current goes into the body as a whole. The vitalometer is so constructed as to give the operator a "signal buzz" when the current is flowing through the instrument. This faint "buzz" is a distinct advantage to the operator since it eliminates the possibility of testing a tooth and concluding it to be non-vital only to discover that the electric current is not flowing through the instrument.

Technique.—The bipolar electrode instrument such as the vitalometer, being the type in most general use, the following suggestions for the technique of making a vitality test will be found helpful.

If the instrument being used for the vitality test is functioning as it should, the success or failure in vitality testing depends entirely upon the operator's knowledge of vitality testing and his technique.

It is best to test anterior teeth on the incisal edge or by straddling the incisal edge with the bipolar electrode. This last method would place one point on the labial and the other on the lingual. Posterior teeth are best tested on the occlusal surface by placing the electrode in the sulci and allowing one point of the electrode to touch one of the cusps.

Before placing the electrode on the tooth the operator must make certain that the tooth to be tested is sufficiently moist. Moisten

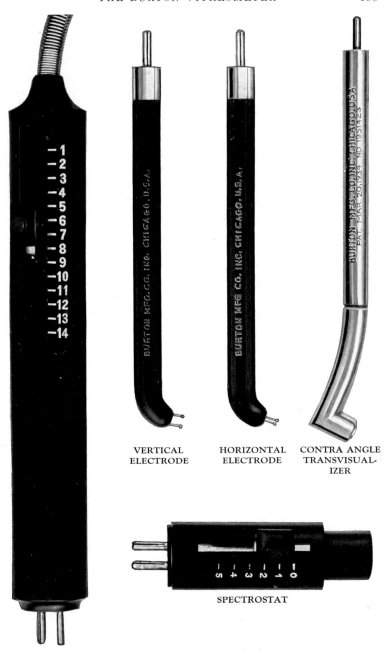

VERTICAL   HORIZONTAL   CONTRA ANGLE
ELECTRODE   ELECTRODE   TRANSVISUAL-
                                   IZER

SPECTROSTAT

Fɪɢ. 237   Fɪɢ. 238
Fɪɢs. 237 and 238.—The Burton Vitalometer for testing vitality of pulp
and Transilluminator for complementing roentgenological examinations.

the tooth to be tested with saliva, but bear in mind the saliva dries rapidly when the mouth is open. If difficulty is experienced in maintaining constant moisture, spreading a very thin layer of tooth-paste on the tooth will give a constant, even moisture that will not dry quickly. Care must be taken to see that the tooth-paste is spread only on the tooth to be tested and does not carry over to the adjacent teeth or to the gums. It is very important to have moisture when testing, since moisture acts as the conductor and without a good conductor for the current the responses are obtained from the patient only by the use of very high voltage. Ample moisture will bring about response at very low voltages, which is to be preferred.

In placing the electrode on the tooth be certain you have good contact. Press the electrode firmly to the tooth to be certain of good contact. Good contact is necessary to obtain early responses.

Start with the instrument set for the lowest voltage. If no response is obtained do not increase the voltage; rather move the electrode slightly to another point on the tooth and try again with the low voltage. Then if no response is obtained increase the voltage to the next step and again place the electrode at two or three different places on the tooth. Remember that the resistance of the tooth varies at different parts and by moving the electrode from place to place on the tooth you will discover the site of least resistance and in that way obtain a response with the least amount of current.

There is nothing known which does not have its limitations, and the most outstanding limitations of testing the pulp for vitality by using electric current are:

Multi-rooted teeth where the pulp is vital in one root and non-vital in another. A response can be obtained from the vital root.

Teeth with large deposits of secondary dentine are very slow to respond to the current. On such teeth it is possible to obtain no response at all unless contact and moisture are carefully watched and checked.

Teeth with large metallic fillings can be tested by taking care to dam the tooth off from adjacent teeth if the metal touches the adjacent teeth. If the tooth being tested contains an occlusal filling it can be tested by placing one electrode point on the metal and one on the tooth, thus straddling the margin of the filling. If the filling touches the soft tissue the electrode points must contact only the tooth structure, not the metal.

Crowned teeth cannot be tested without removing the crown unless it is shallow enough to retract the gingival margin, thus allowing the electrode points to touch only the tooth. Teeth containing putrescent pulps have been known to give a vital reaction due to the moisture acting as a conductor of the current. Do not expect to be able to diagnose diseases of the pulp with electric current. Thus far little progress has been made in that direction. It is possible to test vitality.

The Thermal Test.—The thermal test for vitality of teeth is practised most commonly by the application of ice to the tooth in question. The procedure: A small piece of ice is placed in a towel or some other material which will absorb the water as the ice melts; the ice is then held in contact with the tooth for a few seconds. If no response, the ice is placed in contact with the corresponding tooth on the opposite side of the mouth and the time in which the tooth responds noted. By comparison, it is possible to test fairly accurately the vitality of the pulp.

Another thermal test is placing a hot instrument to the surface of a tooth, but today this method is considered rather poor procedure. And another seldom used test is by the use of an ethyl chloride spray, this necessitating the isolation of the tooth with the rubber dam, and has been discountenanced since the simpler methods have been utilized.

Roentgenologists should be minutely posted and keep thoroughly informed as to all systems for adequate tests of tooth vitality; and for this purpose, no treatise can be recommended more highly than the chapter devoted to the subject in Prinz's Dental Materia Medica and Therapeutics.

Transillumination (Fig. 238).—In the routine examination of the oral cavity, transillumination can be applied as a supplement to roentgenology and as an aid in disclosing some of the more incipient or elusive conditions. It must not, however, be used with the idea that it will check with the roentgenogram, and without a full knowledge of its limitations. Shadows or opaque areas are found under transillumination, correctly applied, only when there exists a localized morbid change in the soft tissue. This so-called shadow is explained as being due to deoxygenation of the red blood corpuscles in the area of stasis. Where the condition is general, or where free drainage exists, a shadow will not be present.

Finding of these shadows indicates infection which may or may not be corroborated by the roentgenogram, depending upon whether or not there is any bone or hard tissue destruction or rare-faction. A diagnosis cannot be made from transillumination findings alone.

The transilluminator will aid in uncovering cavities and caries which may or may not be disclosed on the roentgenogram. Bite-wings are often of little value in disclosing cavities in the anterior teeth and transillumination of the anteriors may disclose them.

Tiny cavities are often disclosed under transillumination which exist just below the gingival margin. These are best found after the patient has been given a prophylaxis because calculus deposits often make such tiny cavities difficult to discern in routine examination.

Transillumination can be used to disclose the presence or recurrent decay under synthetic porcelains and at the margins of ordinary fillings and inlays, but its use should not be intended to replace the roentgenogram. A good transilluminator is always of value for specific mouth illumination for general oral examination by direct vision.

INTERPRETATION.

The outstandingly important phase of modern medicine and modern dentistry, of course, is diagnosis; and that is "the sum total and correlation of the history, the clinical findings, and the results of the various specialized methods of examination." When less is comprehended in our examination of conditions we fail in making a diagnosis.

Since it is usually neglected until local discomfort is caused, a focus of infection may be very difficult to diagnose; and to discover and diagnose these local foci when systemic disease occurs requires alert and thorough examination. Hasty, superficial conclusions are undependable; the only method whereby sufficient information and knowledge may be attained is through painstaking search, the elimination of every uncontributing factor, and the reduction of all possible conditions to the basic pathological cause.

After the roentgenogram has been produced and confirmed to be sufficiently clear and without distortion, we come to the most important phase of dental roentgenography. That is the interpretation of the roentgenogram which, combined with our clinical findings and history of the case, enables us to render a diagnosis and proceed with the proper treatment.

The history of the patient becomes valuable in many interpretations. The roentgenogram (Fig. 239) was interpreted by a rather capable practitioner as indicating a cyst, with surgical procedure contemplated. While the interpretation was manifestly inaccurate by reason of the appearance of the surrounding bone structure, inquiry would have developed that the removal of an impacted maxillary canine had created the condition.

It is utterly impossible to interpret a roentgenogram unless we have an exact knowledge of the normal anatomy of the area presented in the roentgenogram, and it is often just as utterly useless even to make a roentgenographic examination if a snap diagnosis is made before such examination is made. For example, a typical

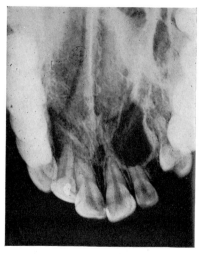

Fig. 239.—Radiolucent area caused by the removal of the maxillary canine but interpreted as a cystic condition.

illustrative case is as follows: A dentist found a gold shell crown on the maxillary right first molar of a patient suffering pain, and ordered a roentgenographic examination. The result perturbed him because it failed to show a condition he presupposed would appear in the first molar. Ignoring the apparent condition in the second premolar (Fig. 637), he sent the patient back with directions for another roentgenogram that would represent the condition he suspected in the first molar.

Actually the first molar was normal. The cause of the pain was a large carious condition under the filling in the second premolar.

But the dentist had carelessly overlooked this in the first roent-genogram simply because he had already predetermined the diag-nosis and thereby had closed his perceptive faculty to any other possibility.

This presents only one of probably thousands of such cases where the lesions was diagnosed prior to the roentgenographic examination, and the moral is: Stop, look and observe before an interpretation is given. Be not too hasty in concluding the existence of conditions from mere clinical appearances.

The diagnosis of chronic periapical disease processes depends upon the history, the symptoms, the clinical examination, and the roent-genographic examination. Quite often errors in diagnosis are observed due to lack of coördination in these various factors or to failure correctly to interpret roentgenographic findings.

"The roentgenogram never lies. When it is thus accused, the operator is reading into it something that is not there or missing something that is there. Of course, from a film alone, a operator can say that in such a location the film shows up darker than normal, or lighter, but that is not interpretation. Interpretation is the determination of the histologic, anatomic, and pathologic con-dition present in any given area, and this requires more than a roentgenogram." (Thomas.)

Chronic periapical lesions often exist in the absence of clinical signs and symptoms. Then, roentgenographic examination becomes the only means of diagnosis. Even in the absence of symptoms, a periapical rarefied area as shown in the roentgenogram does mean usually that the disease of some kind is present, unless, as might some-times happen, the exposure has been made so shortly after an opera-tion that the rarefied area has not had time to become obliterated.

The claim has been made that these areas of rarefaction shown by the roentgen-ray are non-infective in the absence of pain and local symptoms, and may simply represent the results of previously exist-ing disease that has been cured. In other words, it is contended that they contain harmless scar tissue. While conceding this pos-sibility in a small number of cases, the persistence of such a rarefied area for any length of time without decreasing in size is sufficiently justifiable evidence that a disease process is going on; otherwise the area would become smaller and be replaced by new bone. There is abundant postoperative evidence that these areas of rarefaction disappear and are replaced by new bone unless infection remains.

Postoperative pathological findings so strongly support the view that these rarefied areas shown by the roentgen-ray are active foci of disease in most cases, that it is the wisest course to regard them as diseased until proven healthy; and this rule should govern particularly and especially in cases of invalids. It is a much more serious matter to leave a potential source of systemic infection than to sacrifice a healthy tooth.

ILLUMINATION.

The proper illumination of the roentgenogram for the purpose of interpretation is very important. The light should be soft and

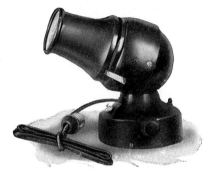

FIG. 240.—Victor Mabeescope which supplies excellent illumination for the interpretation of roentgenograms.

diffused, its intensity being controlled by means of a rheostat. Ordinary daylight will not serve; it is too difficult to control.

Preferably the source of light should be from the blue daylight Mazda lamp, the light passing through "flashed opal" glass, and controlled by a rheostat, enabling the operator to regulate the intensity of the light. This is quite necessary, as all roentgenograms are not of the same density. By means of the rheostat the operator may cut down the intensity of the light for thin negatives; while for the denser negatives he may increase the intensity of the light. The flashed opal glass, because of its even distribution or diffusion of the light allowing the roentgenogram to be illuminated over its entire area, has the advantage over ordinary ground glass.

In the selection of equipment, the operator should be vigilant to secure the apparatus that carries out these principles. (Figs. 194 and 240.)

Particularly attractive to dentists are the new operating cabinets, with their upper section well equipped with two conveniently placed diagnostic view boxes. A four-degree rheostat provides for the variation of light, and a lead-lined film safe protects and stores unused film. (Fig. 241.)

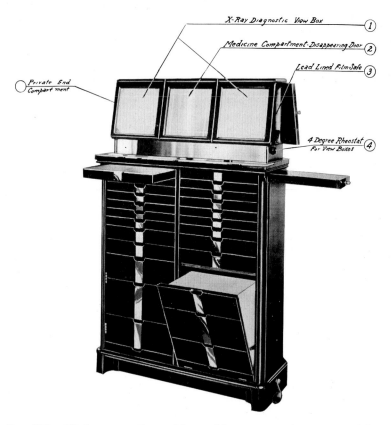

FIG. 241.—Modern operating cabinet with upper portion converted into a diagnostic view box and film safe.

CHAPTER VIII.

NORMAL ANATOMICAL LANDMARKS OF THE TEETH AND JAWS AS SEEN IN THE ROENTGENOGRAM.

In interpreting roentgenograms, no words of explanatory terminology are used more or with greater meaning than are the expressions "radiopaque" and "radiolucent." For the immediate purpose, it will suffice it to mention they apply respectively to the lighter areas and the darker areas appearing on the films, the lighter areas being spoken of as *radiopaque*, the darker areas as *radiolucent*.

The teeth lie in sockets and are attached to the alveolar process by the alveolo-dental periosteum. The alveolar process is composed of cancellated bone (Figs. 242 to 245), which appears in the roentgenogram as a fine interlacing network. The alveolar process is that part of the jaw bones which supports the teeth and is composed of compact and cancellous tissue, arranged in its external contour and internal structure to meet most efficiently the stresses transmitted during mastication.

The relation of opposing teeth, the length of the cusps, the different degrees in the axial angles of the mandibular and maxillary teeth, the influence of the excessory factors involved in mastication, and all other agents—pathologic or otherwise—which affect individual bones or the osseous system in general, are as indelibly imprinted on the structures of the alveolar process as are environmental influences on other bones of the body.

Cancellous bone is homogenous with compact bone as structural material, and differs from it mechanically only in that it possesses less strength in proportion to its density than does compact bone. Cancellous bone is found where the chief function of the bony structure is to transmit tensile and compressive strains. Thus does Koch describe it, and he mentions that "the trabeculæ carry these stresses in the most economical manner, according to the well recognized principle of mechanics that the most direct manner of transmitting stress is in the direction in which the stress acts."

On roentgenograms can be seen transitions from cancellous to compact bone around individual teeth which represent the changing types of stress to which each part has been subjected. Most of the

(207)

varying densities shown on the film can be explained by the physiologic law that "the thickness and closeness of spacing of trabeculæ in bone vary directly with the intensity of the stresses transmitted by them."[1] A closer spacing of trabeculæ around a tooth is evidence of an increase in the stress of mastication, while a wider spacing is characteristic of a disuse atrophy of the part. These conditions are not necessarily due to infection or inflammation but are, funda-

FIGS. 242 to 245.—**Important Anatomical Structures Surrounding the Teeth.**

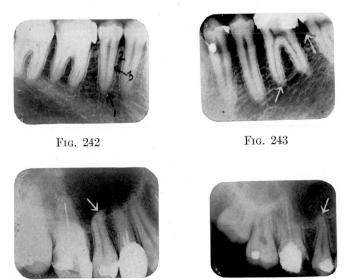

FIG. 242   FIG. 243

FIG. 244   FIG. 245

FIG. 242.—1, the lamina dura; 2, the bony septum separating the sockets of the teeth; 3, the alveolo-dental periosteum. Any deviation of these three anatomical landmarks usually indicates some pathological involvement.

FIG. 243.—Showing the cancellated bone of the alveolar process; the lamina dura; alveolo-dental periosteum; and a loss of the apex of the bony septum between the first and second molars.

FIGS. 244 and 245.—Showing the lamina dura passing around the roots of the maxillary molar and premolar teeth, establishing the fact that the roots of the teeth do not communicate with the maxillary sinus.

mentally, changes in bone due to physiologic stimulation or a lack thereof. The tooth sockets are lined with a thin plate of dense bone, which show in the roentgenogram as a fine radiopaque line passing

[1] Koch, J. C.: Laws of Bone Architecture, Am. J. Anat., **21**, 177, 1917.

around the tooth. (Figs. 244 and 245.) It is the lamina dura. Between the lamina dura and the tooth itself will be found a radiolucent space, this representing the alveolo-dental periosteum. (Fig. 243.) These lines and spaces are important landmarks in the interpretation of roentgenograms, as their absence or deviation usually means the presence of some pathological condition.

LANDMARKS OF THE MAXILLA.

At varying distances above the apices of the first and second incisors is found the inferior meatus of the nose, or the nasal fossa,

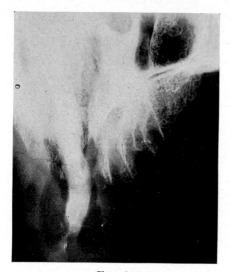

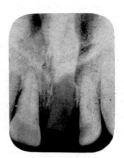

Fig. 246   Fig. 247

Fig. 246.—Roentgenogram of an edentulous maxilla showing the nasal cartilage extending anterior to the alveolus in the incisor region.

Fig. 247.—The very dense radiopaque area extending through the center of the film and down between the left first incisor and the right second incisor in the space formerly occupied by the right first incisor is the nasal cartilage.

which appears in the roentgenogram as two large radiolucent areas divided by a broad radiopaque line representing the septum of the nose. (Figs. 256 to 258.) The nasal fossa has often been mistaken for cystic cavities in the bone.

In examinations of the anterior region of the maxilla, we must know that in some patient the cartilage of the nose may be so

14

dense and prominent as to absorb more rays than usual, resulting in a radiopaque shadow appearing superimposed over this area, as seen in Figs. 246 and 247. Lack of knowledge of this condition has often caused misinterpretation of the film.

THE NASOPALATINE CANALS.

There is a slight depression in each nasal fossa about 2 cm. posterior to the inner wall of the nostril and in juxtaposition to the nasal septum. The depression leads into a small funnel-shaped canal lined with mucosa, which is a continuation of the lining of the inferior nasal meatus. This tube of mucous membrane, the nasopalatine canal, runs caudalward and converges with its fellow

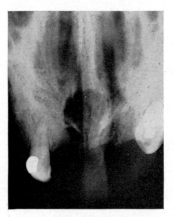

FIG. 248.—Median cyst. Probably a residual dental root cyst in the median line which is very often interpreted as a median cyst. It may be, however, the result of the obliteration of both extremities of the nasopalatine canals.

of the opposite fossa toward the nasal septum, descends vertically and passes through the Y-shaped incisive foramen in the hard palate.

The right and left nasopalatine canals may join the anterior palatine canal and form a common channel; but more commonly each retains its individuality. The canals end in the palate on either side of the incisive pad.

The nasopalatine canals are remnants of the wide communication between the nasal and oral cavities found in early fetal life. Occasionally, in the adult, the canals lead to a direct communication between the oral and nasal cavities. In the vast majority of cases, however, the canals are obliterated and represented by impervious cords of epithelial cells continuous with the epithelium of the mouth and the nose. In some cases it is difficult to find any remnant of the canals.

If we recall that the nasopalatine canals in the embryo connect the inferior nasal meatus with the oral cavity, we can readily understand why cells arising from them may communicate with the nasal fossa or the oral cavity in later life. And if both extremities of the nasopalatine canal become obliterated, and the center remains open, it could readily give rise to a median cyst. (Fig. 248.)

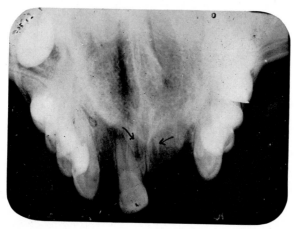

Fig. 249.—An occlusal roentgenogram of the anterior portion of the palate showing the nasopalatine canals on both sides of the median suture.

The nasopalatine canals very often are of such size that they appear in the roentgenogram as radiolucent lines on either side of the anterior palatine foramen. (Fig. 249.)

On the palatal surface just behind and between the first incisor teeth is found the incisive fossa. (Fig. 250.) This contains foramina carrying blood-vessels and nerves from the nose through the anterior palatine canal, which is the canal communicating between the oral and nasal cavities. (Fig. 253.) In roentgenograms of the anterior teeth, this fossa is frequently seen as a radiolucent area above and between the maxillary first incisors, and, when in close relationship to the roots of the teeth, might be mistaken for a rarefied area due to infection. (Fig. 256.)

In a roentgenogram of the second incisor, and sometimes in cases of the first incisor, the apical region of the first incisor may appear

FIGS. 250 to 252.—**The Median Palatine Suture.**

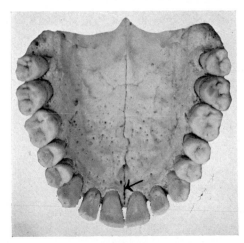

FIG. 250

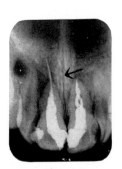

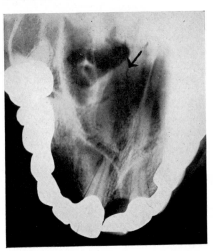

FIG. 251   FIG. 252

FIG. 251.—Palatine surface of the maxilla, showing the median palatine suture running anterio-posterior.

FIGS. 251 and 252.—Radiolucent line running anterio-posteriorly is the median suture.

FIGS. 253 and 254.—**Anterior Palatine Canal and Foramen.**

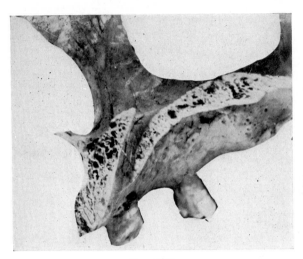

FIG. 253

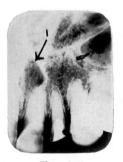

FIG. 254

FIG. 253.—Section of the maxilla through the sagittal plane, showing the anterior palatine canal passing between the nasal fossa and the oral cavity.

FIG. 254.—Radiolucent area over right maxillary first incisor.

FIGS. 255 to 258.—**Anterior Palatine Canal and Foramen.**

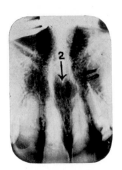

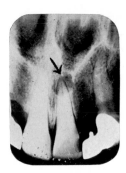

FIG. 255   FIG. 256

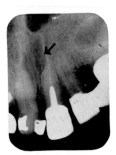

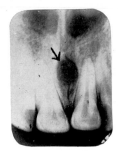

FIG. 257   FIG. 258

FIG. 255.—The same case as seen in Fig. 254, the radiolucent area is between the maxillary first incisors, evidencing how this area representing the foramen can be shifted on the film merely by a deviation in the angulation at which the tube is placed.

FIG. 256.—Anterior palatine foramen over right maxillary first incisor.

FIG. 257.—Anterior palatine foramen slightly superimposed on the right maxillary first incisor.

FIG. 258.—Very radiolucent foramen, due to sharp angulation. When extremely radiolucent areas appear, there usually appears accompanying an evident foreshortening of the teeth. This results from the angulation of the rays being nearly parallel with the long axis of the anterior palatine canal.

superimposed upon the anterior palatine foramen (Fig. 256), and this result might impress the uninitiated as an indication of a pathological condition. But such a conclusion may be radically wrong.

An inaccurate angulation in taking the first incisor may project the radiolucent area over the apex of either maxillary incisor (Fig. 259) because the direct rays will have passed through the tissues in a line that superimposes the roots of the first incisors over the anterior palatine foramen. (Fig. 254.) Unless the interpreter were keen to realize the angle at which the roentgenogram was taken, an erroneous interpretation would follow.

To confirm any interpretation of roentgenograms so appearing, the rays should be directed perfectly parallel to the sagittal plane,

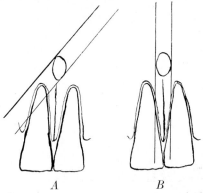

A B

Fig. 259.—A, central rays directed obliquely to the sagittal plane, causing the anterior palatine foramen to be superimposed upon the apical third of the root of the first incisor, as seen in Fig. 254. B, central rays directed parallel to the sagittal plane, causing the anterior palatine foramen to take its proper position between the first incisors (Fig. 255).

and the proper angulation attained. Then, if the radiolucent area moves back to a position above and between the first incisors, and in the sagittal plane (Fig. 255), which is the normal position, we deduce that no pathological condition exists and that the seeming pathological area was produced by the anterior palatine foramen.

The degree of radiolucency depends upon the vertical angle of the direct ray and the angle of the anterior palatine canal in the maxilla. (Fig. 253.) If the rays are parallel to the long axis of the canal, the shadow cast will be darker (Fig. 258) than it would be if the rays were directed perpendicular to the long axis of the canal, because at the former angle the rays pass down the canal and are not absorbed, thus striking the negative with a greater intensity. (Fig. 262.) When directed perpendicularly, the rays pass through a considerable portion of alveolar process, and are extensively absorbed.

The anterior palatine canal, varying so greatly in length, size and shape, presents a problem when interpreting films of this region. As the canal passes upward and backward through the palatal plate of the maxilla (Fig. 253), it opens into the floor of the nasal fossa on either side, and very often the foramen at the nasal terminus of the canal is much larger than the anterior palatine foramen;

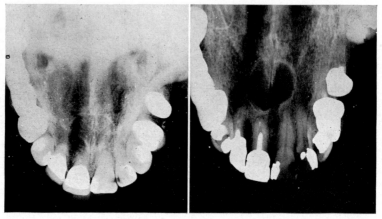

Fig. 260   Fig. 261

Figs. 260 and 261.—The anterior palatine canal appearing rather large and radiolucent.

Fig. 260.—The roentgen-rays directed perpendicular to the plane of occlusion show the area to be in direct communication with the anterior teeth, and not as radiolucent as it appears in Fig. 261.

Fig. 261.—The rays were directed at an angle of 65 degrees to the plane of occlusion and show the canal and foramen more radiolucent and have the appearance of being divided, one-half being on each side of the septum.

and as the canal enters the nasal fossa at an angle, the foramen is not a circle but is more egg-shape in that its anterior-posterior dimension is greater than its lateral dimension. In the roentgenographic examination this condition must always be kept in mind. Sometimes we find rather large radiolucent areas, which are confusing because of our conception of the anterior palatine foramen as rather small; but knowing that we have the entire canal to consider, we realize the radiolucent area may be of any size. Because of its size and position this area is very often misinterpreted in the roentgenograms as a median cyst. (Figs. 260 and 261.)

In roentgenograms of the anterior teeth, frequently a radiolucent line appears, extending posteriorly from the border of the alveolar process in the median line of the maxilla. This line is the median palatine suture. (Figs. 250, 251 and 252.)

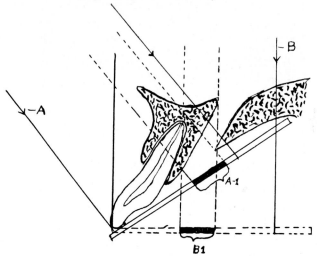

Fig. 262.—*A*, proper vertical angulation of the central rays; the rays passing through a considerable amount of bone and through the short axis of the canal producing a radiolucent area on the film at *A*-1, as seen in Fig. 256. *B*, rays directed perpendicular to the plane of occlusion and passing through the long axis of the canal, causing a foreshortening of the teeth and the canal reproduced at *B*-1, appearing in the roentgenogram as a very radiolucent area, as seen in Fig. 258.

Passing along the outer surface of the skull, we come to the region of the third molar, and here, on the outer surface we find a number of anatomical landmarks of deepest importance of interpretation. They are:

1. The tuberosity of the maxilla, which articulates with the tuberosity of the palate (Fig. 254), and which appears in the roentgenogram as normal cancellated bone curving upward at the posterior border of the maxilla. (Fig. 271.)

2. The hamular process of the sphenoid bone. It is a hook-like projection at the apex of the internal pterygoid plate, around

which plays the tendon of the tensor palati muscle.   (Fig. 263.)
In the roentgenogram it appears as a radiopaque hook-like projection extending downward and backward from the tuberosity of the

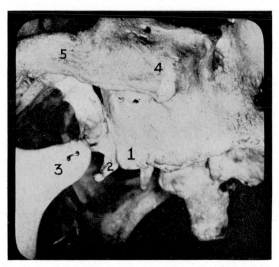

Fig. 263.—1, the tuberosity of the maxilla; 2, the hamular process of
the sphenoid bone; 3, the coronoid process of the mandible; 4, the malar
bone; 5, the temporo-malar suture.

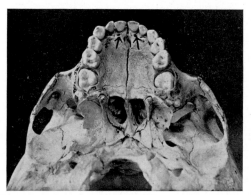

Fig. 264.—Accessory foramina found sometimes in the maxilla.

maxilla. (Figs. 270 and 271.) It has more than once been mistaken
for a fragment of the maxilla, the interpreter mistakenly concluding
it to have been fractured during the removal of the third molar.

3. The coronoid process of the mandible. This appears as a large triangular-shaped process anterior to the sigmoid notch. It passes downward and forward when the mouth opens (Fig. 263), and is seen in the roentgenogram as a radiopaque triangular area posterior to the tuberosity of the maxilla. (Figs. 271 to 275.) It

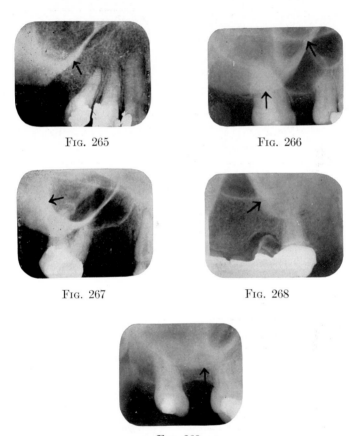

FIG. 265

FIG. 266

FIG. 267

FIG. 268

FIG. 269

FIGS. 265 to 269.—The malar bone in its varying forms and densities.

may, however, appear to be superimposed on the maxilla (Fig. 274) or extend as far forward as the first molar. (Fig. 273.)

4. The malar bone and its zygomatic process. (Fig. 263.) This appears in the roentgenogram as a large radiopaque area over the molar region and is often very troublesome because of the difficulty in securing the detail desired, due to the shadows caused by the

malar bone. (Figs. 265 to 269.) This difficulty may be overcome to a great degree by the employment of Le Masters' technique, as related on page 86.

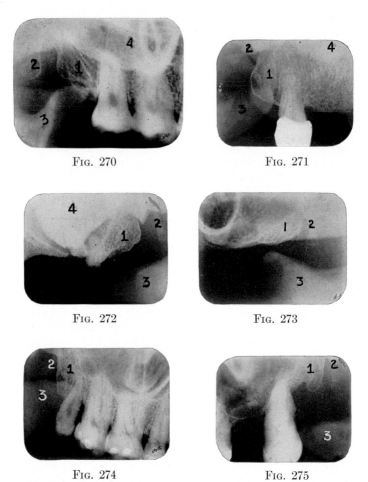

Fig. 270   Fig. 271

Fig. 272   Fig. 273

Fig. 274   Fig. 275

Figs. 270 to 275.—Illustrating the normal anatomical landmarks as seen in the region of the maxillary third molar. 1, the tuberosity of the maxilla; 2, the hamular process of the sphenoid bone; 3, the coronoid process of the mandible; 4, the malar bone.

5. The temporo-malar suture. (Fig. 263.) This forms the attachment of the zygomatic process of the malar bone with the zygomatic process of the temporal bone. It passes downward and backward

from the superior border of the zygoma, and appears in the roentgenogram as a radiolucent line. (Fig. 276.) This, too, must not be mistaken for a fracture.

6. On the palatine surface in the molar region are found the posterior palatine canal and foramen. (Fig. 250.) It is rarely seen in the roentgenogram, though occasionally it shows as a radiolucent area in the wall of the maxillary sinus, in close relation to the palatal roots of the molar teeth.

7. In many roentgenograms a rarefying area indicated in the palate often confuses the interpreter as to whether such an area signifies a cyst or a sinus. Accurate determining of this doubt is important; and, seemingly, the surest way of distinguishing and determining is to locate positively the contiguous inner wall of the maxillary sinus and the outer wall of the nasal fossa. (Figs. 312 to 319.)

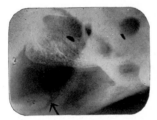

Fig. 276.—Temporo-malar suture.

THE MAXILLARY SINUS.

Certain parts in the anatomy of the maxillary sinuses must be adequately understood by the dentist to enable him to render an intelligent opinion in numberless cases of suspected disease changes in the upper dental arch. The maxillary sinus, the largest of the paranasal sinuses, in addition to being subject to structural and pathological variations found in the other sinuses, presents a series of special problems by reason of the relationship it bears to the teeth. With the prominence of the theory of focal infection as a source of systemic disease have come many harmful procedures by both dentist and physician because both have been groping in the dark.

The sinus is present at birth; it enlarges until, at about the age of six years, it has descended to the level of the middle nasal meatus; by the time of puberty it has expanded inferiorly until its floor is opposite the floor of the nose. In adult life it is typically found to be below this level and in the alveolus. The expansion sometimes continues into the palate and into the tuberosity behind the upper third molar. These extensions are significant clinically. Arrest of development through inherited factors or through disease may cause considerable alteration in the roentgenologic appearance. Variations in the principal skull diameters may so alter the shape of the maxillary sinus that different individuals may have sinuses of the same shape but of totally different radiographic appearance.

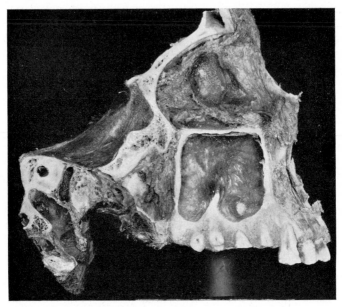

Fɪɢ. 277.—Septum present in the floor of the maxillary sinus. (Cryer.)

Comprehensive studies of the maxillary sinus by the anatomist and by the rhinologist from their respective points of view have been at our disposal; but their observations present a veritable maze to the dentist whose interest lies mostly in a more definitely limited phase of these studies. Clinical observations have been collected to permit an advanced evaluation of information pertaining to the maxillary sinus, and it behooves every dentist to acquire an intensive knowledge of the relative size, the conformation, the location of the sinuses, and the physiological, anatomical and pathological conditions pertaining to them and to the structures and the regions contiguous to them. The dentist must know from the angle of the roentgenologic examination how to interpret the shadows that may develop on the film, how to recognize the distinguishing points whereby the normal structure may be differentiated from the pathological change.

We do know the maxillary sinus as a cavity of varying dimensions, always present in the maxilla, its extension or enlarging process accompanying the growth of the face.

At birth, it exists merely as a slit-like indentation upon the outer wall of the nasal fossa; for at this period of life the maxilla is

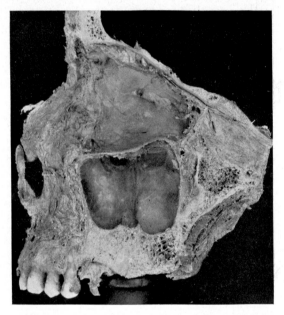

FIG. 278.—Showing the floor of the maxillary sinus divided by two septa. (Cryer.)

made up almost entirely of the alveolar process, the sockets of the unerupted teeth being almost in contact with the orbital plane of the maxilla.

Of course we observe its presence and the phenomena of its growth even earlier; for Schaeffer even indicates that about the seventh day of fetal life the maxillary sinus begins to grow from the evagination of the mucous membrane of the floor or lateral wall of the ethmoidal infundibulum, forming a primitive pouch. Sometimes there forms two such pouches, the fusion of which probably explaining the rather rarely met double adult maxillary sinus, each part of which has its independent ostium.

By the end of the first year of life we observe the maxillary sinus developed in width to reach below the orbit, although not beyond the position of the infra-orbital canal; and by the twentieth month it develops further posteriorly to the position of the rudimentary first permanent molar.

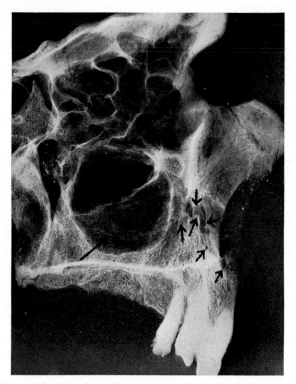

Fig. 279.—A lateral view of a maxillary sinus, showing it to be rather small and circular. The walls in this particular sinus are very thick on all sides. Close observation will show the posterior-superior alveolar artery traversing the sinus wall and its anastomosis with the anterior-superior alveolar artery forming a loop anterior to the sinus, as depicted by the arrows.

This early growth is related in historical and chronological detail so that a better understanding may be had of the later, maturer developments.

In the third and fourth years there is a very conspicuous growth in width, which progresses increasingly thereafter until, at the seventh years, we note an average width of 18 mm., an average height of 17 mm., an average length of 27 mm.

With children, seemingly, the size, the growth of the maxillary sinus progresses proportionately with the progress of age and dentition, although, until the teeth erupt and the alveolar process develops, little space avails for this sinus. But we know the process goes on, developing downward until, about the age of puberty, or about the time practically all permanent teeth save the third molar have erupted, the floor of the sinus is on the level with the floor of the nose.

The largest of the paranasal sinuses, the adult maxillary sinus, resembles in general a three-sided pyramid, lies laterally to the outer side of the nasal fossa, and occupies a greater part of the maxilla, its walls of varying thickness. (Figs. 277, 278 and 279.)

The lining of the sinus is a delicate vascular muco-periosteal layer, a ciliated epithelium containing mucous glands, its deeper portion serving as a periosteal covering of the cavity. This lining is continuous with the lining membrane of the middle meatus through the ostium maxillare.

The median wall or base is directed toward the nasal fossa, the apex of the pyramidal-shaped cavity lying at the zygomatic process of the maxilla. The upper or orbital wall is often modeled by the ridge containing the infra-orbital canal; the anterior wall is toward the face and is varyingly impressed by the canine fossa. Although often reduced by the extensions of the sinus into the adjacent alveolar process, the posterior-inferior wall is normally the thicker.

In studying conditions connected with the sinuses, the dentist must have in mind that they vary greatly in size in different individuals, and quite often in the two sides of the face of one person (Fig. 280); and also that they become modified by local enlargements so as to lose the typical pyramidal appearance.

Zuckerkandl[1] discusses these extensions of the maxillary sinus as (1) alveolar, (2) palatine, (3) zygomatic and (4) infra-orbital.

Because of its great dental significance, we add to that classification still another: the tuberosity extension. (Batson.)

As presented by Zuckerkandl, the alveolar extension is produced by the hollowing out of the alveolar process. (Fig. 281.) Occurring after the age of puberty mostly, and observed most prominently in the region of the first molar, the sinus often extends into the bifur-

[1] Der Anatomie der Nasenhöle, Leipzig, 1893.

15

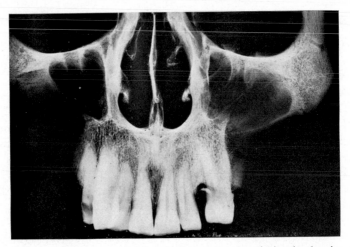

FIG. 280.—A vertical section of a skull showing a variation in the size and shape of the maxillary sinuses in the same individual.

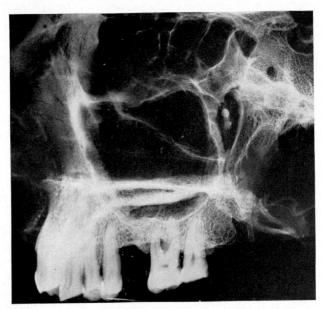

FIG. 281.—*Alveolar extension of the maxillary sinus.* Showing lateral view of the maxillary sinus with a decided alveolar extension. The floor of the maxillary sinus is decidedly below the floor of the nose in the region of the second molar. See Figs. 291 and 292.

cation of the roots of the first molar. (Fig. 284.) Roentgenograms made after extraction of the first molar show the sinus extending further into the alveolar process, sometimes almost to the crest of the alveolar ridge. (Figs. 282 to 294.)

And it is extremely important that this particular extension be recognized as such, for the uninformed may interpret it as a cystic area or some other pathological lesion. (Fig. 285.)

The palatine extension is the designation given to the excavation of the floor of the nasal fossa by the extension of the alveolar process between the plates of the hard palate. (Figs. 295 and 296.)

This would show more in the anterior third of the palate, and may extend over to the median line of the palate, appearing in the roentgenogram (Figs. 297 and 298) as a continuation of the anterior portion of the maxillary sinus.

As first suggested by Ennis, 1930, it may be differentiated from a cystic area by following the outline of the typical Y that develops in the roentgenogram as the line of the inner wall of the sinus reaches the region of the first premolar.

For the clearer indication and surer interpretation of this, the occlusal film seems to serve the better; and because this palatine extension is less common than the alveolar extension, extreme caution must be used to guard against misinterpretations of this condition.

The designation of infra-orbital extension covers the encroachment of the sinus into the frontal process of the maxilla.

While seemingly of less importance than the alveolar extension and the palatine extension, it is very necessary that the operator be able to interpret the infra-orbital extension clearly, for sometimes it forms a typical pocket between the infra-orbital canal and the inner wall of the sinus. Failure to recognize this condition may be serious; for when making posterior-anterior views of these sinuses the pocket may cast a shadow over the nares and the ethmoidal sinus which, improperly interpreted, may be taken for an abnormal lesion that would lead to an unjustifiable surgical procedure with results that may prove dire.

Omitting comment on the zygomatic extension because of its minor significance to the dentist, we come to consideration of the tuberosity extension.

While the posterior-inferior wall of the sinus is usually the thickest (Fig. 281), yet, in numerous examinations, we discover the sinus extending so into this wall as a tuberosity extension that it causes a

Figs. 282 to 289.—**The Maxillary Sinus, Its Septa, and Alveolar Extension.**

Fig. 282.—An alveolar extension of the maxillary sinus showing the sinus dipping down into the bifurcation of the roots of the second maxillary molar. The sinus also dips into the alveolar process in the region of the extracted first molar but with a residual root of the first molar in position.

Fig. 283.—The maxillary first molar having been extracted, the maxillary sinus has extended into the alveolar process until there remains only a very thin wall of bone between the sinus and the oral cavity.

Fig. 284.—Septum of the maxillary sinus over the second premolar, dividing the maxillary sinus into two parts, the posterior portion of the sinus extending down into the bifurcation of the roots of the first molar.

Fig. 285.—Maxillary sinus, alveolar extension in the region formerly occupied by the first molar. This condition exists after extraction of a tooth such as the first molar in Fig. 284.

Fig. 286.—Maxillary sinus, alveolar extension between the molar and premolar teeth.

Fig. 287.—A very thin septum in the maxillary sinus.

Fig. 288.—Septum of the sinus directly over the second premolar.

Fig. 289.—Septum of the sinus directly over the second premolar. There is a diagnostic wire in the premolar, but it does not extend beyond the apex of the tooth.

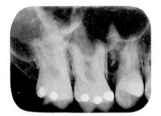

FIG. 282

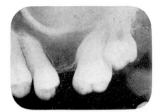

FIG. 283

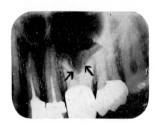

FIG. 284

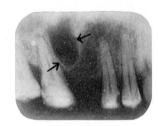

FIG. 285

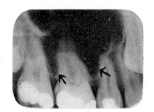

FIG. 286

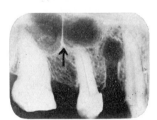

FIG. 287

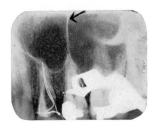

FIG. 288

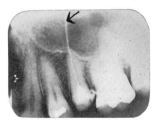

FIG. 289

FIGS. 290 to 294.—**The Maxillary Sinus, Its Septa, and Alveolar Extension.**

FIG. 290.—Maxillary sinus, alveolar extension to the border of the alveolar process under the bridge.

FIG. 291.—Maxillary sinus, the floor of which is on the border of the alveolar process. This is not entirely due to an alveolar extension of the sinus, but to an extensive absorption of the alveolar process.

FIG. 292.—Showing decided alveolar extension of the maxillary sinus with a small septum in the sinus in the region of the second premolar, causing the sinus to appear as though it had a decided elevation in its floor.

FIG. 293.—Indicating the loss of the three maxillary molars and a decided alveolar extension of the maxillary sinus, showing a very small amount of bone remaining between the maxillary sinus and the oral cavity.

FIG. 294.—A decided alveolar extension of the maxillary sinus in the region of the missing maxillary first molar. There is also a definite area of granulation tissue with a rarefying osteitis over the apical region of the premolar.

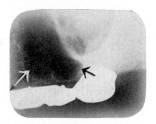

FIG. 290

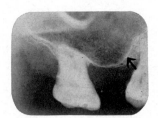

FIG. 291

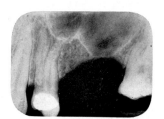

FIG. 292

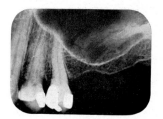

FIG. 293

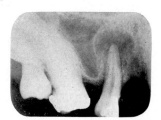

FIG. 294

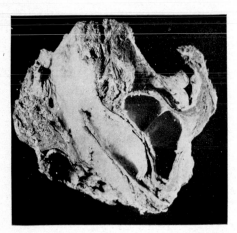

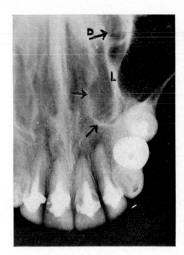

FIG. 295

FIG. 296

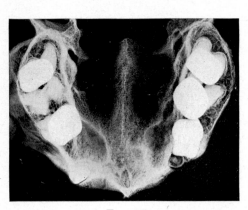

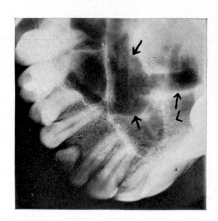

FIG. 297

FIG. 298

FIG. 295.—An anatomical specimen cut on the plane of the floor of the nose showing the maxillary sinus extending over toward the median line of the head. Also two septa dividing the sinus into three compartments.

FIG. 296.—Roentgenogram of specimen shown in Fig. 295 showing the maxillary sinus extending toward the median line in the palatal plate. The extension is greater on one side than on the other.

FIG. 297.—A palatine extension of the maxillary sinus showing the sinus extending toward the median line from the lateral wall of the nose, designated *L* in the roentgenogram. *D* in roentgenogram is the lacrimal canal in the lateral wall of the nose.

FIG. 298.—The palatine extension of the maxillary sinus, marked by arrows. The lacrimal canal has been slightly distorted and appears as an elongated radiolucent shadow (*L*). The typical "Y" formation dividing the maxillary sinus from the nasal fossa may be observed over the apical region of the canine. The palatine extension may be seen anterior to this region and superimposed over the nasal fossa.

(232)

thinness not only of the posterior-inferior wall but also the supporting structure of the third molar and, sometimes, of the second molar.
(Fig. 299.)

Recognition of this condition is impressively important, and
especially so when it becomes necessary to extract the teeth of this
region. Because of the thinness of the alveolar plates and the posterior wall of the sinus (Figs. 300 to 303), the plates may fracture
and come away with the teeth, leaving a large opening in the alve-

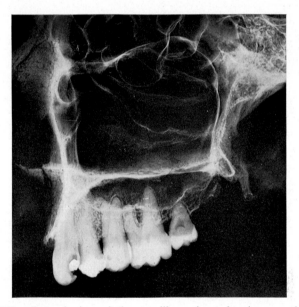

Fig. 299.—Lateral view of the maxillary sinus showing a rather large
sinus with extensions in practically all directions. The tuberosity extension
is rather marked, making the posterior-inferior wall rather thin.

olar process with only the muco-periosteal lining separating the
sinus from the oral cavity.

Thus, later, after the tissues have been restored, there would be
practically no alveolar ridge upon which a denture could be constructed. There would remain merely a flat plane. But with a
thorough understanding of this tuberosity extension, teeth may be
removed surgically without a great loss of their bony support.

When it becomes necessary to perform an alveolectomy in an
edentulous mouth having a bulbous tuberosity of the maxilla, it
is critically essential that we ascertain the presence or absence of

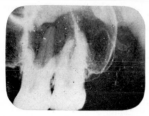 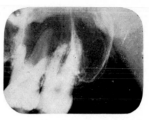

FIG. 300.—A decided tuberosity extension, revealing a septum over the third molar, and the posterior wall of the sinus very thin.

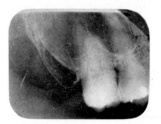 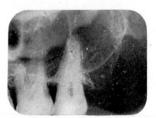

FIG. 301.—Tuberosity extension of the maxillary sinus, extending decidedly posterior to the third molar.

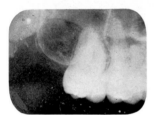 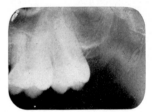

FIG. 302.—Tuberosity extensions of both the right and the left maxillary sinus which were diagnosed as cysts.

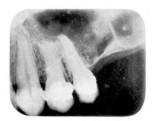 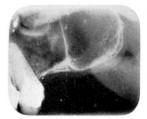

FIG. 303.—Tuberosity extension of the maxillary sinus. The molar teeth have been extracted, leaving a very thin plate of bone between the maxillary sinus and the oral cavity.

any tuberosity extension of the sinus; for otherwise the operator may find himself making an opening into the maxillary sinus.

Especially might be noted cases where the maxillary sinus seems particularly large, a condition due to an extreme hollowing out of the sinus in all directions. (Fig. 299.) This creates a condition of thinness of the sinus walls, with extension markedly developed; and it should be obvious that no attempt to operate in the molar or premolar regions should be made without a most thorough roentgenographic study.

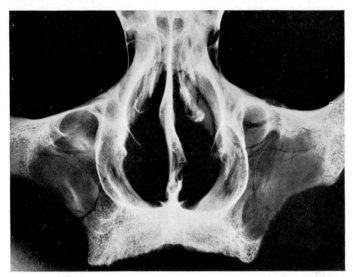

Fig. 304.—Vertical section of a skull revealing an excessive bulging of the lateral walls of the nose. The palatal process in this particular specimen is rather thick. Note the nutrient canals in the walls of the sinus.

The mere enumeration of these anatomical variations of the maxillary sinus should impress the dentist with the high requirements of information and knowledge relative to the entire region, and that less than a thorough knowledge spells danger.

While not nearly so important from the angle of dentistry as are these enlargements which govern our operative procedure, nevertheless we must not ignore the distinguishing cases where less developed or more contracted conditions of the sinus are manifested. Many and varied causes conduce to bring about these conditions. They may be due to imperfect absorption of the cancellated bone on the floor of the sinus; or by reason of a secondary thickening of the sinus walls; or from an unusual depression of the canine fossa; perhaps from imperfectly erupted teeth; or from excessive bulging of the lateral nasal wall (Fig. 304); or from improper aëration of the sinus during growth and development due, as mentioned by Shea, of Memphis, to a nasal disease in the maxillary ostium.

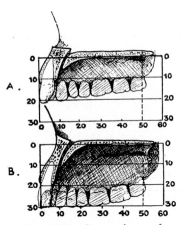

FIG. 305.—Comparison of a well-developed palate (*A*) with one (*B*) showing a high degree of contraction. Both specimens have been cut on the sagittal plane; both are arranged on a horizontal base passing along the plane of the hard palate. (Keith.)

In the interpretation of roentgenograms we must not overlook the least of the variations that are manifested in the maxillary sinus; the differences discovered among even normal sinuses are so great that cases of abnormal sinuses charge the operator and the interpreter with responsibility of knowing to the greatest degree the veriest detail of the anatomy of the maxilla and its surrounding structures.

We cannot possibly recognize fully the variations in the anatomical appearance of the maxillary sinus without having clearly in mind the relationship between the floor of the sinus and the floor of the nasal fossa.

While, about the age of puberty, the floor of the sinus is on the level with the floor of the nasal fossa, from that period the floor of the sinus descends below the floor of the nasal fossa. The degree

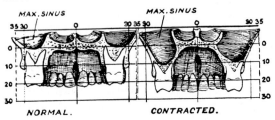

FIG. 306.—Coronal sections of a normal and of a contracted palate. The sections were made distal to the first molar teeth and are viewed from behind. (Keith.)

of descent depends upon the degree of the hollowing out or pneumatization of the alveolar process of the maxilla.

Sir Arthur Keith[1] reports a series of measurements showing that the nasal cavities in cases of contracted palate are not more shallow than usual, but that their floors, formed by the hard palate, are at normal levels, something happening to cause the alveolar bone to grow and expand more in a vertical direction and less in an horizontal direction. (Fig. 305.)

From another series of measurements he concludes that one feature of these sections is seen in the downward expansion of the maxillary sinuses which, in the normal palate, descend to the level of the palatal plane but which, in the contracted palate, descend

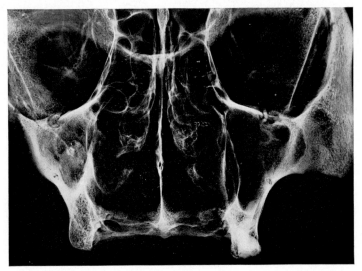

FIG. 307.—Vertical section of a skull revealing an excessive bulging of the lateral walls of the nose and resorption of the alveolar process, causing the floor of the sinus on the right to be on a level with the floor of the nose, while on the left the floor of the maxillary sinus is considerably above the floor of the nasal fossa.

10 mm. below this plane, so that in the abnormal palate the direction of growth of the alveolar bone, and the expansion of the maxillary sinuses, progress more vertically than in the normal palate. (Fig. 306.)

We observe also that the degree of arching of the hard palate, affecting, as it does, the floor of the nose, has some bearing on the relationship of the floor of the sinus to the floor of the nasal fossa.

[1] The Growth of the Jaw, Normal and Abnormal in Health and Disease. The Dental Board United Kingdom.

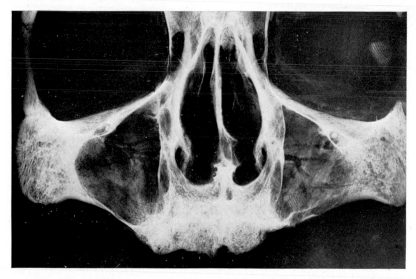

Fig. 308.—Vertical section of the skull revealing a very thick palatal plate with the floor of the nose a considerable distance above the floor of the maxillary sinus. Note: The nutrient canals passing through the anterior wall of the maxillary sinus on either side.

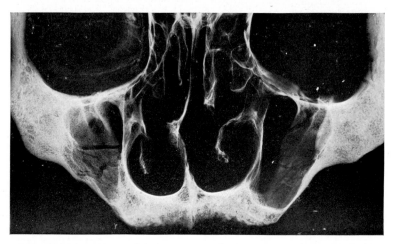

Fig. 309.—Vertical section of a skull revealing the resorption of the alveolar process causing the maxillary sinus to recede. The floor of the nasal fossa is practically on a level with the floor of the maxillary sinus.

With the resorption of the alveolar process following the loss of teeth in later years (Figs. 307 to 309), we find a process of recession of the maxillary sinus, the greater the resorption, of course, the greater the recession; so that when the alveolar process is completely resorbed we find the floor of the maxillary sinus again on the level with the floor of the nasal fossa about as it appeared at the age of puberty. (Fig. 310.)

In considering the relationship of the maxillary sinus to the teeth, we know immediately that this relationship cannot be con-

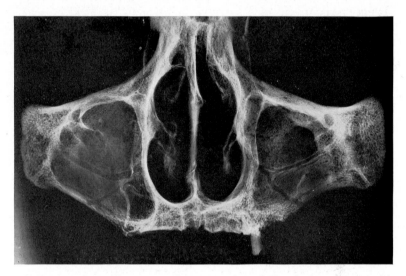

Fig. 310.—Revealing a complete resorption of the alvolar process with the floors of the maxillary sinuses and the nasal fossa being practically on a level. Note the radiolucent nutrient canals in the walls of the maxillary sinus.

stant. The variations in the size of the sinuses and the variations in the teeth tell that.

The cancellated bone between the roots of the teeth and the floor of the sinuses varies in thickness in different individuals; and if the cancellated bone be thin, the roots of the teeth form elevations on the floor of the sinus, these elevations contributing to form recesses.

The extension of the sinus into the alveolar process presents the direct communication between the roots of the teeth and the mucous membrane of the sinus. This intimate relation between teeth and sinuses must ever be in mind, and with a clear mental picture of the sinus, you will appreciate the exact number of teeth bearing direct relationship must be inconstant, depending primarily upon the size of the sinus.

Occasionally we find the canine tooth in direct relationship, although not nearly so often as the premolars. In fact, the three molars are in intimate, vital relationship with the floor of the sinus in the vast majority of cases observed.

Frequently the walls of the maxillary sinus are noticed to be uneven, recognition of which anatomical condition is important. It may be no manifestation of a pathological lesion. The irregulari-

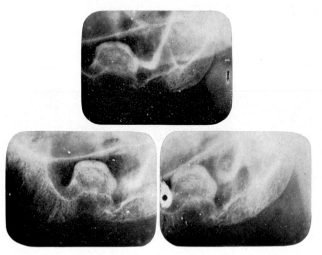

FIG. 311.—Large septum traversing the maxillary sinus anterior-posteriorly.

ties or uneven spots consist of ridges or crescentic projections of varying sizes and proportions, which occasionally are replaced or followed by septa. (Figs. 277, 278, 300, 303.)

The smaller ridges need not be considered of deep consequence, but the large ones that tend to form pockets and recesses of different depths within the cavity may not be disregarded.

The septa sometimes divide the sinus into two cavities and, forming at various angles and heights, are anatomical warnings of which the operator must beware when interpreting roentgenograms of this region and when treating conditions subsequently. (Fig. 311.)

Theory suggests that the larger septa might be a development from the two primary pouches often discovered in the early stage of life, the intervening wall disappearing in part to leave the large septa we see among adults. But the chief explanation of these osseous projections on the wall of the sinus is probably the unequal resorption of the bone during the development of the sinus, the sinus developing along the line of least resistance.

Very often we find blood-vessels within the septa. This may

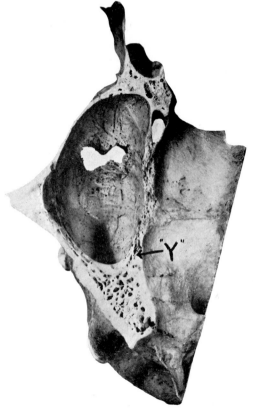

Fig. 312.—Specimen cut on plane of the floor of the nose, showing the nasal fossa extending anterior to the maxillary sinus, thus forming the typical "Y." See Figs. 314 to 318.

indicate that, as the sinus developed and extended, the bone containing these vessels offered more resistance to the process of pneumatization.

Unfamiliarity with the anatomical structure of the maxilla has been the cause of irremediable errors because of the failure to recognize minute details of the maxillary sinus and its anatomical variations.

16

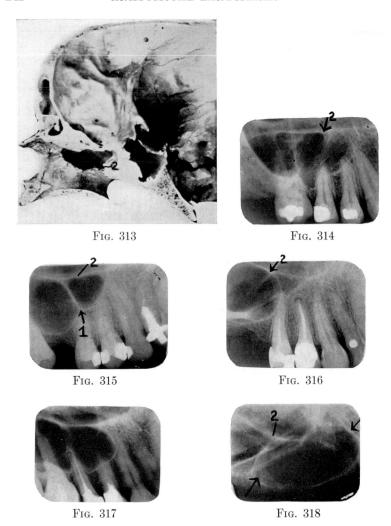

FIG. 313   FIG. 314

FIG. 315   FIG. 316

FIG. 317   FIG. 318

FIG. 313.—2, the area of line shown in the roentgenogram, dividing the maxillary sinus from the nasal fossa.

FIGS. 314 to 317.—Fig. 314, innerwall of sinus extending antero-posteriorly, the anterior wall leaving the inner wall at 2, forming a typical "Y," the nasal fossa extending farther forward.

FIG. 315.—The maxillary sinus completely divided by a septum (1), while the wall of the sinus (2) extends further forward to form the "Y."

FIG. 316.—The typical "Y" dividing the maxillary sinus from the nasal fossa.

FIG. 317.—The typical "Y."

FIG. 318.—The typical "Y" appearing (2), the area designated by the arrows being a cyst.

Thousands of cases must be examined and studied before we attain fully a realization of these variations; and they may be classified only after the slightest distinctions among these variations can be detected; for, like the historian, the dentist needs a wide knowledge of the past before he can interpret the present.

One of the most invariable of the anatomical structures of the maxilla is the inner wall of the maxillary sinus which, as you know, is the inner wall of the nasal fossa. Very irregular, it is formed anteriorly by the nasal process of the maxilla with the posterior margin, of which the lacrimal bone articulates; the middle portion

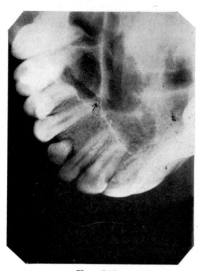

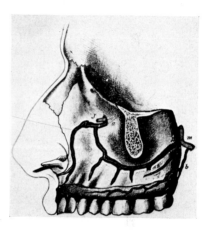

Fig. 319   Fig. 320

Fig. 319.—Occlusal roentgenogram of the palate disclosing very clearly a typical "Y" formed by the nasal fossa extending anterior to the maxillary sinus, as illustrated in the anatomical specimen, Fig. 312.

Fig. 320.—The arterial arcade of the upper teeth. (After Zuckerkandl.) *m*, the internal maxillary artery; *a*, anterior-superior alveolar (dental) artery; *p*, posterior-superior alveolar (dental) artery; *b*, buccinator artery.

of the wall is formed by the lateral mass of the ethmoid bone above the inner surface of the body of the maxilla, the inferior turbinate bone at the lower end, and, posteriorly, by the vertical plate of the palate bone and internal pterygoid plate.

This inner wall separates the nasal fossa from the sinus; and we discover the floor of the nasal fossa extending far more anteriorly than the floor of the sinus; and, as the inner wall of the nasal fossa extends forward, the anterior wall of the maxillary sinus swings outward laterally, then posteriorly, as the outer wall of the maxillary sinus. (Fig. 312.)

Where the anterior wall of the sinus swings away from the outer walls of the nose, a typical Y is formed. (Fig. 312.) In the crotch of this Y is cancellated bone which supports the premolar, canine and incisor teeth.

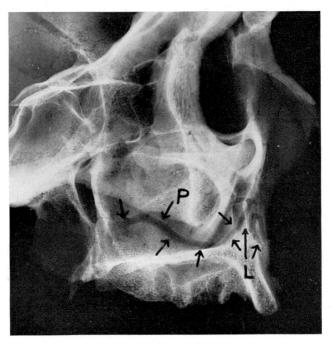

Fig. 321.—The arterial arcade or arterial loop. Arrows point to the path of the posterior-superior alveolar artery which, in this particular case, is rather large, the artery passing forward and anastomosing with the anterior-superior alveolar artery. *P*, posterior-superior alveolar artery; *L*, loop in the region of the infra-orbital foramen showing the anastomosis of the posterior-superior alveolar artery with the anterior-superior alveolar artery.

This Y, therefore, becomes the most differential diagnostic landmark in the interpretation of intra-oral roentgenograms.

The smaller intra-oral films often show the inner wall of the maxillary sinus extending forward as a radiopaque line over the molars and premolars; and this Y formation may be observed as the line reaches approximately the region of the first premolar. (Figs. 314 to 318.)

However, where radiolucent areas here create doubt as to whether it is a normal sinus or a pathological condition, and the typical Y cannot be detected, we should resort to the occlusal film; for with

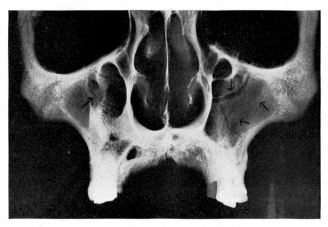

Fig. 322.—Nutrient canals in the anterior wall of the maxillary sinus.

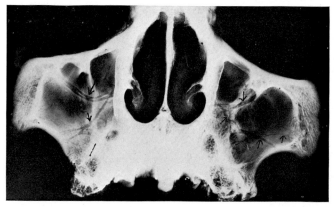

Fig. 323.—Nutrient canals in the anterior walls of the maxillary sinuses, their branches being pointed out by small arrows.

this film we will obtain a general view of the entire region and thus will be able to trace the inner wall of the sinus forward, noticing clearly the Y formation where the floor of the nasal fossa extends anterior to the floor of the maxillary sinus. (Fig. 319.)

Figs. 324 to 331.—**Nutrient Canals of the Maxilla.**

Fig. 324.—Nutrient canal passing downward and forward in the outer wall of the maxillary sinus.

Fig. 325.—A plexus of nutrient canals in the anterior wall of the sinus.

Fig. 326.—Large nutrient canal over the premolars with an infected cyst over the first molar.

Fig. 327.—A plexus of the nutrient canals in the floor of the sinus.

Fig. 328.—A nutrient canal near the crest of the ridge of the maxilla.

Fig. 329.—A nutrient canal making a definite circle between the second premolar and first molar, which may very readily be mistaken for a pathological area.

Fig. 330.—A nutrient canal coming straight down the wall of the sinus and communicating with an inflammatory condition at the apex of the second premolar.

Fig. 331.—Terminal branch of a nutrient canal passing horizontally over the apex of the first and second incisor.

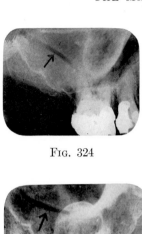

FIG. 324

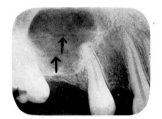

FIG. 325

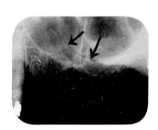

FIG. 326

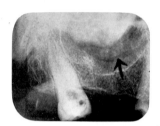

FIG. 327

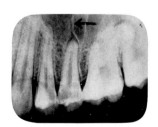

FIG. 328

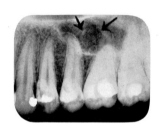

FIG. 329

FIG. 330

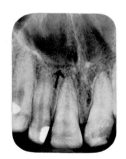

FIG. 331

FIGS. 332 to 337.—**Nutrient Canals of the Maxilla.**

FIG. 332.—A nutrient canal passing vertically between the apical third of the roots of the first and second incisors.

FIG. 333.—Nutrient canal directly over the apex of the maxillary canine.

FIGS. 334, 335, and 336.—Illustrating in the same case the differences of appearance of a nutrient canal superimposed over the apical third of the maxillary canine when roentgenographed from three distinct angles.

FIG. 337.—Nutrient foramen in the maxilla. Note the dense bone found around the canal and foramen. This is the common terminal branch of the posterior superior alveolar artery found in the canine region.

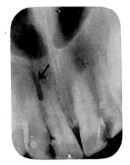 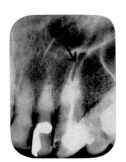

FIG. 332   FIG. 333

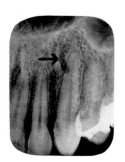 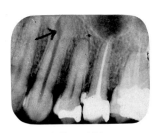 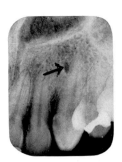

FIG. 334   FIG. 335   FIG. 336

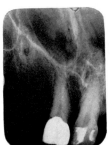 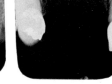

FIG. 337

Once these structures are definitely located, we are in an advantageous position to determine the presence of pathological conditions; and it is appropriate to mention that in the inner wall of the sinus we will generally discover the lacrimal canal as a radiolucent area, which frequently has been interpreted inaccurately as the posterior palatine foramen or as a pathological area.

Proper interpretation of roentgenograms of the molar and premolar area involving the sinus demands also a knowledge of the blood supply and the nerve supply of the sinuses and teeth in that region.

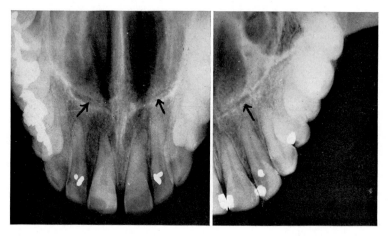

Fig. 338.—Nutrient canals passing forward to the outer anterior wall of the nasal fossa.

Traveling practically the same path are the internal maxillary artery and the maxillary branch of the trigeminal nerve, which supply the maxillary teeth and the muco-periosteal lining of the sinus.

The posterior-superior alveolar artery, a branch of the internal maxillary artery and the posterior-superior dental branch of the trigeminal nerve descends upon the tuberosity of the maxilla, where it breaks up into a plexus. (Fig. 320.)

Branches of both artery and nerve penetrate through small foramen in the bone, supplying the molar and premolar teeth and the mucous membrane of the sinus. They occur in the outer wall of the sinus in a groove, or, more generally, in a rather large bony canal, which we notice in the roentgenogram as a radiolucent line running anterior-posteriorly through the sinus. In some cases this line extends forward with its terminal branches in the nasal fossa near the ala of the nose. (Fig. 321.)

The infra-orbital artery starts with the posterior-superior alveolar artery, passes through the spheno-maxillary fossa and the spheno-maxillary foramen, and traverses the infra-orbital groove and canal with the infra-orbital nerve.

We know the infra-orbital nerve gives off two branches, the

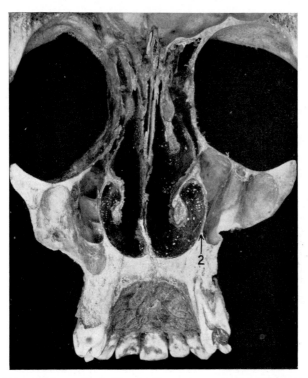

FIG. 339.—Inner wall of the maxillary sinus, dividing the sinus from the nasal fossa. (Cryer.) 2 indicates in the roentgenogram the region which is a great aid in differentiating between the maxillary sinus and cyst formation.

middle and the anterior-superior dental nerves, while the infra-orbital artery gives off the anterior-superior alveolar artery.

It appears that the anterior-superior alveolar artery of the anatomist is more commonly a communicating branch from the infra-orbital artery and the posterior-superior alveolar artery which loops upward near the infra-orbital foramen and receives the communication. (Figs. 320 and 321.)

This anterior-superior alveolar artery, along with the anterior- and middle-superior dental nerves, passes down the anterior wall of the sinus and supplies the canine and incisor teeth and the mucous membrane of the sinus. (Figs. 322 and 323.)

The function of these nerves and arteries is to furnish sensation and supply nutrition. They follow no definite, straight path, but intertwine and bridge across from one canal to another in the bony structure.

The canals will be observed as radiolucent lines in the walls of the sinus. They are sometimes in direct communication with the apices of the teeth, forming over the apical region rather well-defined areas, which should be impressively defined in the mind of the roentgenologist, for too often have these areas been mistaken for pathological conditions. (Figs 324 to 338.)

These canals being so numerous, and the ability to know and specify exactly which one, or which branch of any one, discloses itself in the roentgenogram, being at times difficult if not almost impossible, we employ for all a term that is comprehensive and sufficiently explanatory of their functions, speaking of them as nutrient canals.

THE NASOLACRIMAL CANAL.

At birth the nasolacrimal duct lies about 2 mm. medial to the ventral end of the maxillary sinus and is about 2 mm. in diameter. By the sixth year the maxillary sinus is in fairly intimate relationship with the upper portion of the nasolacrimal duct. By the eleventh year the relationship between the paranasal sinuses and the nasolacrimal ducts is practically that of the adult.

The nasolacrimal canal is a direct continuation of the lacrimal fossa, which is located on the ventro-medial aspect of the orbit. The canal itself is formed by the maxilla, the lacrimal bone and the inferior turbinate bone, the maxilla forming the greater proportions of its boundaries. The canal terminates in a wide-mouth ostium immediately below the attached border of the inferior turbinate on the lateral wall of the inferior nasal meatus.

The diameter of the canal varies from 4 mm. to 7 mm., but is seldom uniform in diameter throughout its length, which varies from 10 mm. to 20 mm.

The plane of direction of the nasolacrimal canal must conform to the type of the facial skeleton. The true plane of the canal is projected in an oblique plane from the lacrimal fossa to a variable point on the medial aspect of the alveolar process of the maxilla, corresponding to the interval between the second premolar and first molar or between the first and second molars, and sometimes between the second and third molars.

The canal courses in the lateral nasal wall between the ventral portion of the middle nasal meatus and the maxillary sinus. The thickness of bone intervening between the maxillary sinus and the nasolacrimal canal varies from a papery thinness to 2 mm. or 3 mm.

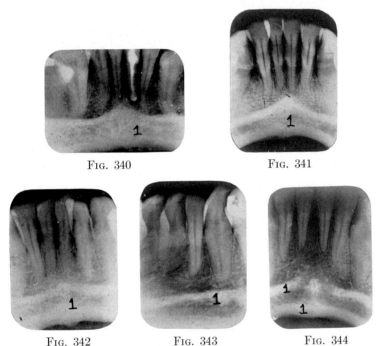

Fig. 340   Fig. 341

Fig. 342   Fig. 343   Fig. 344

Figs. 340 to 344.—The mental ridge. The mental ridge of five different persons, indicating the variation in density and form as seen in the roentgenograms at 1.

In occlusal roentgenograms of the palate the nasolacrimal canal appears as a radiolucent area in the lateral wall of the nasal fossa about the first molar region. (Figs. 297 and 298.)

LANDMARKS OF THE MANDIBLE.

The mandible is a cortical capsule of bone which contains the cancellated bone made up of lamellæ, the arrangement of which makes the cancellated bone have the appearance of a sponge.

(Fig. 242.) The medullated spaces are of different size and must not be diagnosed in the roentgenogram as small cysts.

The principal roentgenographic anatomical landmarks of the mandible, beginning at the symphysis, are:

1. The mental process or mental ridge. This is a dense ridge of bone extending from the symphysis of the mandible to the region of the premolars. As the size of the ridge depends upon the individual, naturally the roentgenographic appearance will vary accord-

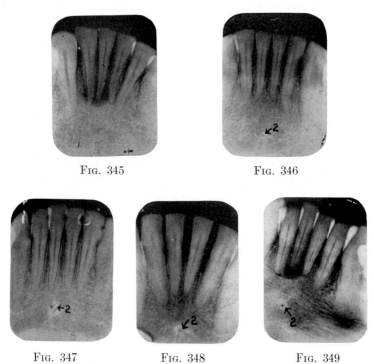

FIG. 345   FIG. 346

FIG. 347   FIG. 348   FIG. 349

FIGS. 345 to 349.—Illustrating the varied appearances of the genial tubercles and the lingual foramen.

ing to individuals. It appears in the roentgenograms as a radiopaque area (Figs. 340 to 344), but differs in density in individuals from an extreme radiopaque area down to that of normal bone, as can be noticed in Fig. 383.

2. The genial tubercles, four in number, two on either side of the median line on the internal surface of the mandible at the symphysis. These appear as a small radiopaque ring with a radio-

lucent area, the lingual foramen, in the center (Figs. 345 to 349), this radiolucent area representing the space between the tubercles.

3. The mental foramen. It lies between and below the roots of the premolars on the external surface of the mandible. In the roentgenogram it appears as a radiolucent area, but as to where it will appear in the roentgenogram (Figs. 350 to 357) depends upon the angulation. It may best be interpreted by following the outline of the mandibular canal.

NUTRIENT CANALS OF THE MANDIBLE.

Roentgenologic examinations of suspected teeth and other parts in the mandible have revealed shadows indicating perfectly normal conditions hitherto mistaken for pathological lesions. They disclose more clearly the ramifications of the mandibular artery and its numberless branches traversing the cancellated structure of the mandible, many of which disclosures had been often inaccurately interpreted as signs of peridental infection.

The mandible holds its place by means of the capsular ligaments and the muscles of mastication, receiving its main blood supply through the mandibular artery. To know the normal anatomy of the mandible comprehends a knowledge of its blood and nerve supply.

Zuckerkandl[1] describes the mandibular artery entering the mandibular foramen, passing forward through the mandibular canal and giving off branches which he designated "interalveolar arteries," and emerging at the mental foramen as the "mental artery." Just before issuing from the mental foramen the mandibular artery gives off an incisive branch which passes forward to supply the region forward of the mental foramen. (Fig. 358.) He describes the blood supply of the teeth and surrounding structures. (Fig. 359.)

The illustration of the blood supply was ingeniously worked out by Batson, 1933, showing more clearly than any hitherto published diagram or description the manifold courses followed by the many branches of the mandibular artery: the mental artery leaving the mandible at the mental foramen, the incisive branch running forward in the mandible to the symphysis, giving off branches passing upward and making their exits through the nutrient foramen on the lingual side of the mandible posterior to the incisor teeth and near the crest of the ridge (Figs. 362, 363 and 364), terminating in the

---

[1] Anatomie der Mundhole, 1891.

FIGS. 350 to 357.—**Mental Foramen.**

FIG. 350.—The mental foramen below the second premolar (3) with the mandibular canal (6) passing back from the mental foramen.

FIG. 351.—The mental foramen between the roots of the premolars (3), the mandibular canal (6) passing downward and backward.

FIG. 352.—The mental foramen below the first premolar (3), the mandibular canal (6) passing forward, downward and backward.

FIG. 353.—The mental foramen over the apex of the first premolar (3), the mandibular canal (6) passing back through the body of the mandible with a granuloma in the apical region of the second premolar.

FIG. 354.—The mental foramen anterior to the first premolar (3), the mandibular canal (6) passing back through the body of the mandible. An accessory canal (5) which is a continuation of the mandibular canal con tinues forward from the mental foramen toward the symphysis.

FIG. 355.—Mental foramen below the second premolar (3), the mandibular canal (6) passing downward and backward, and the accessory branch of the mandibular canal (5) passing anterior to the foramen.

FIG. 356.—Mental foramen (3) below the second premolar, the mandibular canal (6) passing backward from the foramen. There is also a granuloma (7) imvolving the apical region of the second premolar.

FIG. 357.—Mental foramen below the second premolar (3), the area being separated from the apical region of the tooth by the lamina dura.

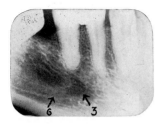

FIG. 350

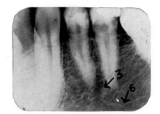

FIG. 351

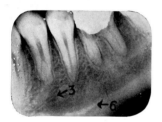

FIG. 352

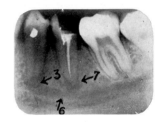

FIG. 353

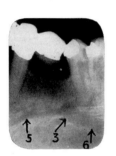

FIG. 354

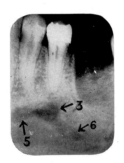

FIG. 355

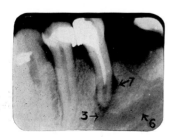

FIG. 356

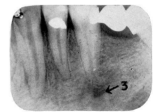

FIG. 357

17

FIGS. 358 to 364.—**Nutrient Canals of the Mandible.**

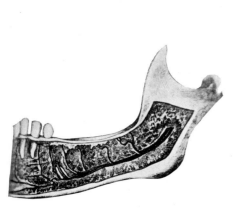

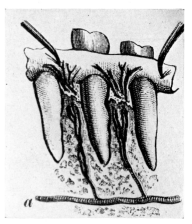

FIG. 358   FIG. 359

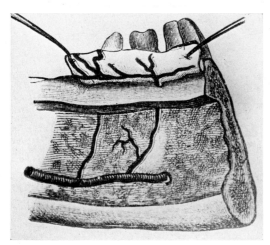

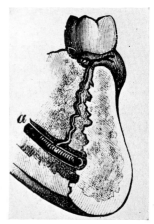

FIG. 360   FIG. 361

FIG. 358.—Mandible with the mandibular artery and its heavier branches exposed. (After Zuckerkandl.)

FIG. 359.—The interdental artery anastomosing with other vessels in the mucous membrane. (After Zuckerkandl.)

FIG. 360.—The interalveolar arteries passing through foramen near the crest of the alveolus and entering the mucous membrane. (After Zuckerkandl.)

FIG. 361.—Large interalveolar artery entering the mucous membrane in the septum between the teeth. (After Zuckerkandl.)

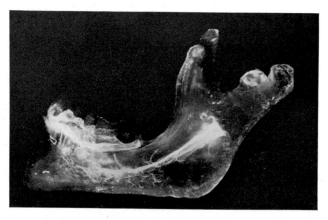

FIG. 362.—An injected and decalcified specimen showing the mandibular artery and its larger branches. The gingival tissue remains on the specimen over the crest of the alveolar ridge showing this tissue to receive its blood supply partly from the mandibular artery. This is a lateral view of the specimen.

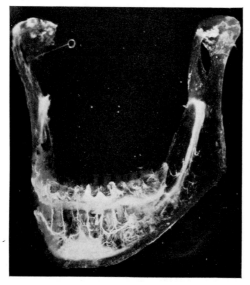

FIG. 363.—A three-quarter view of the specimen (Fig. 362). The mandibular artery with its larger branches in the region of the mental foramen showing the many branches extending vertically toward the crest of the ridge.

gingiva.   Another branch passes through the lingual foramen (Figs.
365 and 366) on the lingual side of the mandible in the region of
the genial tubercle, and anastomoses with the lingual artery.

The mandibular canal through which the artery passes varies
as to its relative position in the structure.   In some cases it may
be observed traversing a line near the lower border of the mandible (Fig. 367), while in other cases it appears near the apical
regions of the teeth (Fig. 368); in some instances it is seen superimposed over the apical third of the roots of the teeth.   (Fig. 369.)
Thus is knowledge of the exact position of the canal important

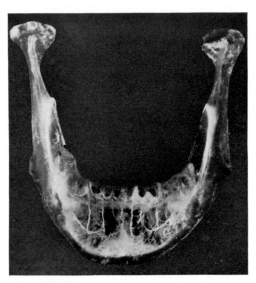

FIG. 364.—The full anterior view of the same specimen (Fig. 362).   We
see the many branches of the mandibular artery extending upward through
the body of the mandible and terminating in the gingiva.[1]

where removal of teeth is contemplated, and particularly when the
third molar is involved.   It appears on the roentgenogram as a
radiolucent area, just as will appear the smaller branches of the
mandibular canal through which pass the lesser branches of the
mandibular artery.   They may be noticed in all parts of the mandible, more numerously in the anterior region.

Although for years these smaller canals have been ignored by
many dentists, the roentgenologist has brought out the important

[1] Specimens shown in Figs. 362, 363 and 364, prepared by Dr. Oscar V. Batson,
Professor of Anatomy, Graduate School of Medicine, University of Pennsylvania.

relation to the entire structural composition of the mandible, and they must be reckoned in considering many phases of operative dentistry. Hirschfeld[1] called them "interdental canals." But as they are not only interdental, being paradental as well, Batson prefers to designate them as "nutrient canals," a term more adequately denoting their functions, for they carry nutrition to the parts by means of the interalveolar arteries.

They appear on the roentgenograms as radiolucent lines passing upward through the body of the mandible, varying in different individuals as to length, width and degree of radiolucency. (Figs. 370 to 383.)

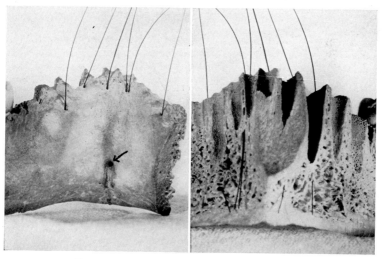

Fig. 365   Fig. 366

Fig. 365.—The lingual surface of the mandible at the region of the symphysis showing the nutrient foramen, delineated by horse hair passing through them, while below, marked by an arrow, we see the lingual foramen.

Fig. 366.—The labial aspect of the specimen (Fig. 365) with the outer plate of the mandible removed, showing the horse hairs passing into the cancellated structure by way of the nutrient canals.

As teeth are lost and resorption of the alveolar process occurs, the nutrient foramen of the mandible approaches the crest of the ridge. Resorption may be so extensive that the outer wall of the nutrient canals may even be lost (Figs. 384 and 385), thus inflicting much discomfort from any artificial restorations.

[1] Interdental Canals, Jour. Am. Dent. Assn., April, 1927.

Figs. 367 to 369.—Nutrient Canals of the Mandible.

Fig. 367.—A lateral view of the mandible revealing the mandibular canal very close to the lower border of the mandible, in the molar region, and looping upward to the mental foramen in the premolar region.

Fig. 368.—Lateral view of the mandible revealing the mandibular canal about halfway between the apical regions of the teeth and the lower border of the mandible. Note that the mental foramen and the width of the canal in this case seem unusually large.

Fig. 369.—A lateral view of the mandible revealing the mandibular canal in very close proximity to the apical region of the second molar, and crossing the apical third of the root of the third molar.

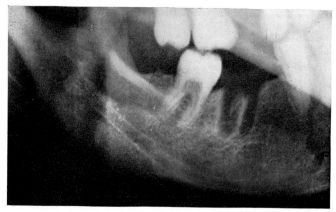

Fig. 367

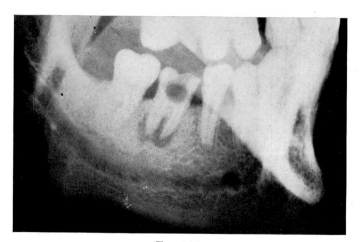

Fig. 368

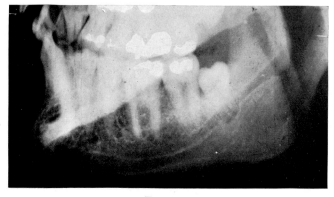

Fig. 369

Figs. 370 to 377.—**Nutrient Canals of the Mandible.**

Fig. 370.—Two rather straight nutrient canals appearing as radiolucent lines in the anterior portion of the mandible between the first and second incisors.

Fig. 371.—A number of rather large nutrient canals in region of the symphysis passing upward through the body of the mandible and terminating at the crest of the ridge.

Fig. 372.—Nutrient canals in an edentulous mandible. The canals being rather short and terminating directly on the crest of the ridge.

Fig. 373.—An edentulous mandible in the region of the symphysis showing the nutrient canals to be much longer than those seen in Fig. 376, but terminating on the crest of the ridge.

Fig. 374.—An edentulous mandible in the region of the mental foramen, revealing the mental foramen near the crest of the ridge, with the nutrient canals rather short and terminating on the crest of the ridge anterior to the mental foramen.

Fig. 375.—The area of the mental foramen, showing radiolucent lines extending upward through the body of the mandible and terminating at the crest of the ridge. These radiolucent lines are the nutrient canals.

Fig. 376.—The nutrient canals appearing as rather long radiolucent lines in the region of the first incisors, which had been extracted.

Fig. 377.—A number of nutrient canals extending upward through the body of the mandible, bridging across and connecting with one another in the region of the mandibular premolars. This particular case had been incorrectly interpreted as a residual root.

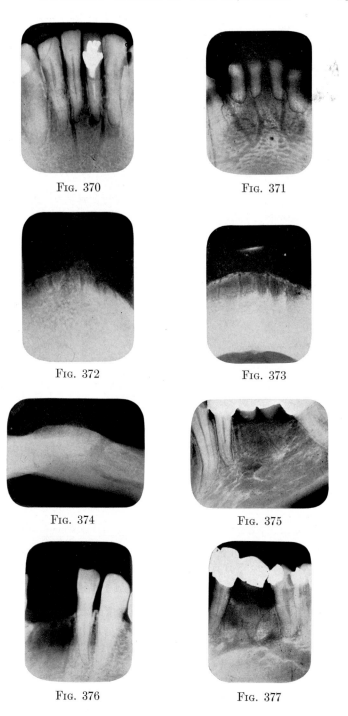

FIG. 370

FIG. 371

FIG. 372

FIG. 373

FIG. 374

FIG. 375

FIG. 376

FIG. 377

FIGS. 378 to 383.—**Nutrient Canals of the Mandible.**

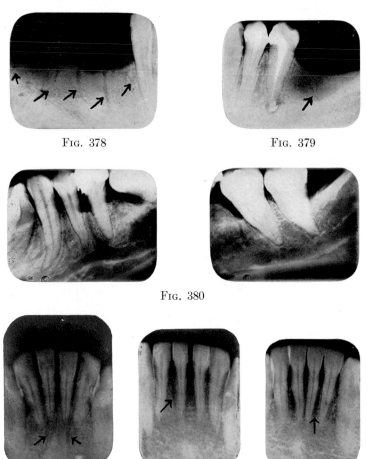

FIG. 378   FIG. 379

FIG. 380

FIG. 381   FIG. 382   FIG. 383

FIG. 378.—The premolar and molar region of the mandible showing nutrient canals with their terminus on the crest of the ridge.

FIG. 379.—Showing a nutrient canal posterior to the mandibular second premolar.

FIG. 380.—The molar and premolar region of the mandible showing a nutrient canal passing upward from the mental foramen between the premolar teeth and terminating at the crest of the ridge. Also a nutrient canal anterior to the second molar, the first molar having been extracted.

FIG. 381.—Nutrient canals found in the mandible between the first and second incisors.

FIGS. 382 and 383.—Nutrient canals varying in length and general appearance.

6. The external oblique line. This is the outer line of the retromalar triangle that passes outward from the mental process and then backward and upward, becoming continuous with the anterior border of the ramus. (Figs. 386 to 392.)

7. The mylohyoid ridge. It commences at the lower part of the symphysis and runs upward and outward to the ramus on the internal border of the mandible. Its greatest development is in the molar region. This, and the external oblique line, both appear of different densities in different types. Therefore, in the roentgenogram they are radiopaque areas, most pronounced in the molar

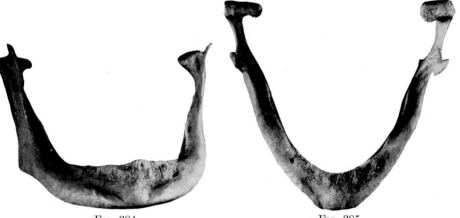

Fig. 384   Fig. 385

Fig. 384.—A mandible, the anterior walls of the nutrient canals completely absorbed, subjecting its nutrient vessels to pressure.

Fig. 385.—A vertical view of the specimen (Fig. 384) showing the nutrient canals to have their terminus on the crest of the ridge. It also shows an amount of absorption had occurred.

region; the mylohyoid ridge, being the lower shadow, often overlaps the shadow of the molar roots. There is also an area of normal bone lying between these two lines, which lines are so radiopaque they tend to indicate the normal bone more decalcified than it really is.

Tooth Development.—The normal development may be clearly portrayed in a series of roentgenograms. Exposures timely made will show the chronology of the processes very vividly. The coronal portion of the tooth is the first to develop, the apical portion being the final stage in the formative process, the entire formation going on within a bony crypt in the jaw. The roentgenogram will show the crypt to surround the entire tooth before eruption; but in erupting, the tooth breaks through and destroys the coronal portion of the

FIGS. 386 to 392.—The External Oblique Line and the Mylohyoid Ridge.

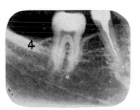 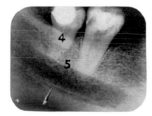 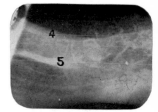

FIG. 386   FIG. 387   FIG. 388

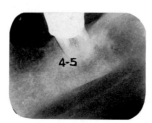 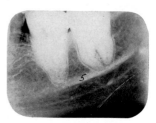

FIG. 389   FIG. 390

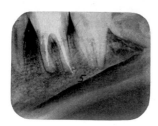 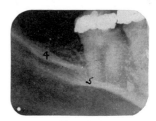

FIG. 391   FIG. 392

FIG. 386.—The external oblique line (4).

FIG. 387.—The external oblique line (4) and the mylohyoid ridge (5).

FIG. 388.—The external oblique line (4) and the mylohyoid ridge (5) practically blending together.

FIG. 389.—The external oblique line and the mylohyoid ridge blended (4–5) together.

FIG. 390.—The mylohyoid ridge (5).

FIG. 391.—The mylohyoid ridge (5) blending into the external oblique line.

FIG. 392.—The external oblique line (4) running into the mylohyoid ridge (5).

crypt. The apical portion of the crypt, however, remains to surround the apical portion of the root until the root has completely calcified. (Figs. 393 to 395.)

FIGS. 393 to 395.—**Tooth Development.**

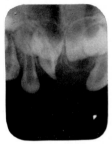
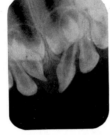
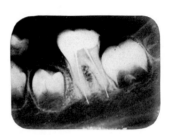

FIG. 393   FIG. 394

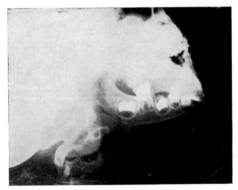

FIG. 395

FIG. 393.—The maxillary first and second incisors in the process of development surrounded by their developmental crypt.

FIG. 394.—The mandibular first molar fully developed. The premolars and second and third molars in the process of development.

FIG. 395.—Lateral view of the mandible beautifully illustrating the bony crypt surrounding a developing tooth.

The development of teeth, while not progressing in any absolutely set manner, may be considered as following a fairly regular evolutionary course, any deviation from which would dictate the requirement of study and treatment.

In normal, healthful subjects the evolutionary phases of dental development may be considered as running along the courses as outlined in the following chart, devised and composed by Dr. Herman Churchill.

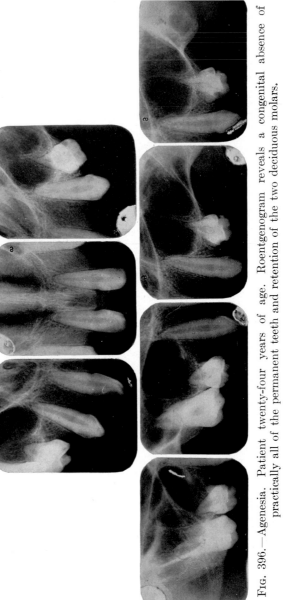

Fig. 396.—Agenesia. Patient twenty-four years of age. Roentgenogram reveals a congenital absence of practically all of the permanent teeth and retention of the two deciduous molars.

EVOLUTIONARY PHASES OF DENTAL DEVELOPMENT.

Deciduous dentition.	1st incisor.	2d incisor.	Canine.	1st molar.	2d molar.	Remarks.
Begins odontogenesis	5th week; length of embryo, 10 mm.					Development and eruption of the teeth in the mandible usually precedes that in the maxilla. Notice exceptions in this table. *Abreviations.* i.u., intrauterine life. maxillary teeth. mandibular teeth.
Calcification begins	4½ mos. i.u.	4½ mos. i.u.	5½ mos. i.u.	5 mos. i.u.	5½ mos. i.u.	
Calcification at birth	½ crown	⅖ crown	¼ crown	Cusps united	⅕ cusps	
Eruption	6-8 mos.	7-9 mos.	16-18 mos.	14-18 mos.	18-24 mos.	
Calcification at eruption	⅓ root	½ root	⅔ root	½ root	½ root	
Calcification ends	2 yrs.	3½ yrs.	3½ yrs.	3½ yrs.	4 yrs.	
Odontolysis begins	4 yrs.	5 yrs.	8 yrs.	6-7 yrs.	7-8 yrs.	
Odontolysis ends	7 yrs.	8 yrs.	12 yrs.	10 yrs.	11-12 yrs.	
Spacing begins	Between 1st and 2d incisors, 5 yrs.		2d incisor and canine, 5 yrs.	1st molar	2d molar	

Permanent dentition.	1st incisor.	2d incisor.	Canine.	1st premolar.	2d premolar.	1st molar.	2d molar.	3d molar.
Odontogenesis begins	5½ mos. i.u.	5½ mos. i.u.	6 mos. i.u.	At birth	10 mos.	4 mos. i.u.	9 mos.	4 yrs.
Calcification begins	2 mos.	2 mos.	4½ mos.	2 yrs.	1½ yrs.	9 mos. i.u.	4 yrs.	8 yrs.
Calcification at birth	....	....	....	....	....	Cusps		
Eruption	6-8 yrs.	7-9 yrs.	10-12 yrs.	9-11 yrs.	11-13 yrs.	5-7 yrs.	13-15 yrs.	16-? yrs.
Calcification at eruption	⅓ root	½ root	⅖ root	⅔ root	½ root	½ root	½ root	½ root
Calcification ends	11 yrs. / 10 yrs.	11 yrs.	13 yrs.	12 yrs.	12 yrs.	12 yrs. / 11 yrs.	15 yrs. / 17 yrs.	19 yrs. / 21 yrs.
Calcification at height of contour	....	....		7 yrs.	7 yrs.			

CHAPTER IX

DENTAL PATHOLOGY IN RELATION TO ROENTGENOLOGY.

FOR the simplest and most comprehensive classification of roentgenographic illustrations and impressions indicating periapical lesions, the profession is greatly indebted to Ivy, whose carefully selected nomenclature, divisions and distinctions have been fairly studiously followed in preparing this particular discussion.

The indispensable basic factor of diagnosis is an assured and accurate understanding of pathology. Without this essential knowledge, it is utterly impossible to give a correct interpretation of roentgenograms of acute and particularly chronic inflammation involving the teeth and their supporting tissues. The diagnostic value of the roentgen-ray in inflammatory processes affecting the teeth and surrounding parts is governed entirely by the variations in the density of the hard tissues as a result of the inflammation. In acute localized infection, the inflammatory process being of too short duration to bring about an appreciable amount of destruction of the bone tissue, the roentgen-ray is of less important value. It is in chronic, long-standing types of infection, or in an acute process grafted upon a chronic one, "exacerbation," that this method of diagnosis finds its greatest field of usefulness.

The roentgenogram being merely the result of the roentgen-ray passing through tissues of various densities and registering on a photographic emulsion, the density of the various tissues through which the rays pass controls the amount of radiation that reaches the photographic emulsion. In roentgenograms of the jaws, the substances depicted in the order of their density, beginning with the densest, and, therefore, appearing the lightest in the negative, are:

1. Metallic crowns and fillings; root-canal fillings; other metals.
2. Enamel of the teeth.
3. Dentine.
4. Cementum.
5. Cortical bone.
6. Cancellated bone.
7. Medullary spaces; canals; foramina in bone; soft tissue.

We have particular terms to apply to the results on the roentgenogram representing the denser or less dense areas or substances through which the rays had been directed.

(272)

When a substances offers little or no resistance to the passage of the rays, a greater intensity of registration upon the emulsion results; and any area of intense registration on the negative will be as a darker area or line, which darker parts we designate as being *radiolucent.*

Rays passing through a normal maxillary sinus, for example, because that cavity is of little, if any, density and, therefore, absorbs little of the rays, strike the photographic emulsion with great intensity, and the result will appear on the negative as a very dark area, a *radiolucent* area.

Radiopaque is the term we apply when the results appear on the negative as the lighter areas or lines, these resulting, as may be easily deduced, from the passing of the rays through tissues of greater density that offer higher resistance and absorb the rays more fully.

If the maxillary sinus be suppurative, that cavity, by reason of the pus content, becomes more dense, and would appear in the negative as a lighter area, a *radiopaque* area; for the increased resistance of the rays, the rays being subject to a greater absorption because of the greater density of material through which it passes, results in a decreased intensity of registration on the film emulsion.

The density of the various tissues and structures determines their transparency or opacity to the roentgen-rays, and thus we designate the transparent quality as *radiolucent,* the opaque quality as *radiopaque.* If any radical changes take place in the tissues, as, for instance, in the case of the normal sinus becoming pathological, a corresponding change would show upon the negative, the normal condition would appear as darker than the subsequent pathological condition, a change from a radiolucency to a radiopacity. And by the same process, where a denser normal structure like a tooth becomes carious and loses substance, we would have a transition from radiopacity to radiolucency on the negative.

Thus the service of roentgenography shows the variations from the normal that demands the highest interpretative faculty and experience accurately to determine and diagnose the different degrees of variation.

Roentgenographic examinations, checked by subsequent extraction of teeth or surgical treatment and followed by histological and bacteriological examinations, show that from a clinical and a pathological standpoint there are in general two types of lesions

18

associated with the teeth where examination by the roentgen-ray is an aid to diagnosis and prognosis. They are:

I. Lesions involving the periapical region of the tooth resulting from infection following death of the pulp.

II. Lesions involving the investing tissues of the teeth—the alveolo-dental periosteum and the alveolar process—not dependent upon the death of the pulp, but in which the infection starts at the gingival margin. Pyorrhea alveolaris, or more correctly, chronic suppurative alveolo-dental periostitis, is an example.

Occasionally is seen another type of lesion, the alveolo-dental periosteal abscess, in which an inflammatory process is set up in the alveolar dental periosteum independently or in the absence of any disease of the pulp, the pulp retaining its vitality or being only secondarily involved. In this type the organisms gain entrace from the gingival margin or from neighboring diseased teeth, or are carried from other parts of the body by the blood stream. (Fig. 486.)

I. PERIAPICAL DENTAL LESIONS.

Lesions of this type are the most important with which we have to treat from a roentgenologic standpoint, because they so often occur in the absence of clinical symptoms or signs, and roentgenographic examination becomes the principal means of diagnosis.

In a majority of the cases the disease results from infection following death of the pulp, the bacteria passing up the root canal and out in to the apical tissues through the apical foramen. Bacteria may also be carried from other parts of the body by the blood stream and lodged in the periapical tissues of pulpless teeth or of teeth containing necrotic pulp tissue. This infection may follow dental caries or inflammation or death of the pulp; it may result from trauma or from artificial devitalization by the dentist. Much has been said as to the part played by various medicinal chemical irritants in the causation of these periapical conditions. Such chemicals might be the starting-point, preparing the way for bacterial infection. But that they alone can induce the reactive process examination of these diseased tissues sometime reveals, continuing and progressing for years, is generally improbable, for we know these chemical agents are limited in the duration of their action by the fact that they cannot perpetuate themselves. It is safer to regard infection by living bacteria as the essential cause of long-standing periapical lesions.

THE THOMAS W. EVANS MUSEUM AND DENTAL INSTITUTE
SCHOOL OF DENTISTRY, UNIVERSITY OF PENNSYLVANIA

DEPARTMENT OF ROENTGENOLOGY

Report on the Roentgenographic examination

of..

Referred by..

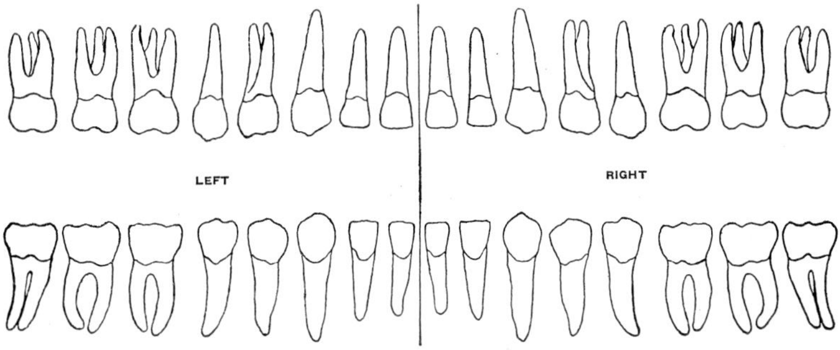

LEFT   RIGHT

Note.—This chart is diametrically opposite to the normal anatomical chart and will be read as the roentgenograms are mounted.

1. Chronic proliferative alveolo-dental periostitis.
2. Chronic rarefying osteitis with granulation tissue.
3. Chronic rarefying osteitis with suppuration.
4. Chronic rarefying osteitis with cyst formation.
5. Alveolo-dental periosteal abscess.
6. Vertical absorption of the alveolar process.
7. Horizontal absorption of the alveolar process.
8. Condensing osteitis.
9. Pulp nodules.
10. Senile dentine.
11. Calcification of the pulp.
12. Root absorption.
13. Hyperplasia of the cementum.
14. Perforated root.
15. Caries.
16. Residual root.
17. Foreign bodies.
18. Fractures.
19. Impactions.

REMARKS:

Date................................Signed...

FIG. 397.—Diagnostic chart for roentgenographic examinations.

Failure on the part of the dentist to observe absolute asepsis in performing root-canal operations is a frequent means of introducing streptococci from the mouth surface into the periapical tissues. The original infection in practically all cases of periapical disease is streptococcal. The access of streptococci to the alveolo-dental periosteum of the apical region in one of the ways mentioned causes a typical inflammatory reaction on the part of the tissues, which is

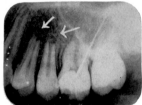 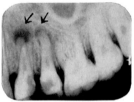

Fig. 398   Fig. 399

Figs. 398 and 399.—Illustrating the difference in appearance between pathological conditions in the apical region and normal development.
Fig. 398.—Roots not fully developed.
Fig. 399.—Rarefying osteitis with granulation tissue.

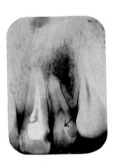 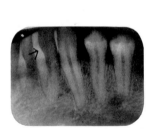 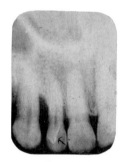

Fig. 400   Fig. 401   Fig. 402

Figs. 400 to 402.—Appearance of enamel tubercles as disclosed in roentgenograms.

Fig. 400.—Enamel tubercles on the lingual side of the maxillary right second incisor.
Fig. 401.—Radiopaque area is caused by the over-lapping or superimposing of the shadow of the mandibular second incisor over that of the first incisor.
Fig. 402.—Enamel tubercle on the lingual side of the maxillary left second incisor.

dependent upon the virulence of the invading organisms and the resistance of the patient. If the streptococcus is of the *hemolytic* type, of high virulence, and the resistance of the patient is low, the inflammation will be acute, and may result in acute abscess formation. If this does occur, with evacuation of the pus under proper treatment, the condition may rapidly subside, with practically no detachment or destruction of the alveolo-dental periosteum, and no appreciable destruction of bone.

In case the invading organism is of the *viridans* type—of low virulence—the inflammatory reaction is apt to be chronic, giving rise to little apparent disturbance, but slowly progressive and proliferative in nature. The first change seen in the alveolo-dental periosteum is a thickening of this tissue, which is infiltrated with various blood elements, but especially polymorphonuclear and small round cells, particularly the latter.

PROLIFERATIVE ALVEOLO–DENTAL PERIOSTITIS.

Etiology.—1. Extension of septic diseases from the pulp.
2. Application of drugs or other irritants.
3. Occlusal trauma.
4. Systemic.

Symptoms.—In acute conditions there is a dull constant pain, relieved by pressure, but returning when pressure is removed. The tooth becomes loosened, but in time returns to its normal firmness. When chronic, pain is slight or may even be absent. Tooth may be permanently loosened.

Roentgenographic Abnormalities.—A slight thickening of the alveolo-dental periosteum about the tooth apex is produced, but without any appreciable loss of bone, which is shown in the roentgenogram by an increased thickness of the normal radiolucent line between the apical portion of the tooth root and the bone. (Figs. 403 to 408.)

CHRONIC RAREFYING OSTEITIS.

Continuous proliferation of the alveolo-dental periosteum takes place at the expense of the bone of the alveolar process, and as proliferation of the round cells occurs, the bone becomes rarefied, and finally destroyed, resulting in chronic rarefying osteitis.

Etiology.—Thickening of the alveolo-dental periosteum at the expense of the alveolar process. With continued proliferation of the round cells the bone becomes rarefied and finally destroyed.

Symptoms.—No clinical symptoms.

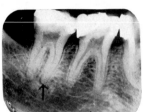 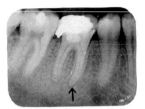

Fig. 403   Fig. 404

Fig. 403.—Thickening of the alveolo-dental periosteum in the apical region of the second molar.

Fig. 404.—Thickening of the alveolo-dental periosteum in the apical region of the first molar.

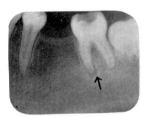 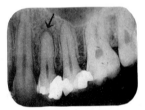

Fig. 405   Fig. 406

Fig. 405.—Thickening of the alveolo-dental periosteum in the apical region of the second molar. The proliferation is more extensive than in Figs. 403 and 404.

Fig. 406.—Thickening of the alveolo-dental periosteum in the apical region of the first premolar. This condition was due to an occlusal trauma.

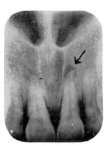 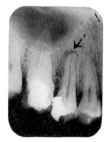

Fig. 407   Fig. 408

Fig. 407.—Thickening of the alveolo-dental periosteum in the apical region of the maxillary first incisor. The condition has advanced to the stage of producing a rarefying osteitis.

Fig. 408.—Thickening of the alveolo-dental periosteum in the apical region of the premolar, due to an occlusal trauma, showing a condition advanced to the stage of rarefying osteitis.

Roentgenographic Abnormalities.—It appears in the roentgenogram as a radiolucent area, the abstraction of lime salts of the alveolar process in the affected area allowing the rays to pass through more readily.

CHRONIC RAREFYING OSTEITIS WITH GRANULATION TISSUE.

Chronic rarefying osteitis leaves this bone space filled with a mass of chronic inflammatory granulation tissue, to which granulation tissue the entirely inaccurate term *granuloma* has been applied; but which term is generally accepted.

Etiology.—Bacterial infection passing out through the apical foramen of a tooth, infecting the alveolo-dental periosteum and causing a chronic inflammatory process to be set up. If the bacteria is of the viridans type of low virulence, the inflammatory reaction is apt to be chronic, producing the granulation tissue.

Symptoms.—No clinical symptoms.

Roentgenographic Abnormalities.—Following rarefying osteitis, the disintegration of the bone is replaced with granulation tissue. The apex of the tooth may project into the bone cavity, be shortened or roughened from irregular absorption of the cementum, or present enlargements due to a hyperplasia of the cementum. In the roentgenogram these lesions are shown as more or less clearly defined radiolucent areas, and vary in size. (Figs. 409 to 432, pages 280 to 285.

The granulation tissue is composed of small round cells, polymorphonuclear and endothelial leukocytes, fibroblasts, capillaries, and fibrous tissue, and sometimes masses of epithelial cells. From this tissue streptococci may be obtained, both by direct smear and by culture. Sometimes the granulation tissue breaks down and is replaced by fluid pus, which fills the bone cavity; or the pus may discharge through a sinus after having become a chronic abscess; or the area of bone disintegration may consist partly of pus and partly of granulation tissue, combining to form a suppurative condition. In the suppurative cases a secondary staphylococcic infection usually becomes superadded to the original streptococcus. Lesions containing fluid pus, however, are in a minority as compared to those containing solely the granulation tissue, and, therefore, the term "chronic abscess" is rarely applicable to the majority of cases of periapical infection.

Figs. 409 to 416.—**Chronic Rarefying Osteitis With Granulation Tissue.**

Fig. 409.—Granuloma in the apical region of the mesial and distal roots of the mandibular left first molar. The buccal-lingual loss of bone is slight. This accounts for the area not being as radiolucent as seen in other cases.

Fig. 410.—Absorption of the apical third of the root of the maxillary right second premolar associated with granuloma. A residual granuloma is present in the region formerly occupied by the first molar.

Fig. 411.—Hyperplasia of the cementum in the apical region of the mandibular right first molar associated with granuloma.

Fig. 412.—Impacted mandibular right third molar associated with a granuloma in the apical region.

Fig. 413.—Perforation at the middle third of the root of the maxillary right canine with an extensive granuloma in that region.

Fig. 414.—Residual granuloma in the region of the maxillary right first premolar.

Fig. 415.—Granuloma on the apex of the lingual root of the maxillary left first molar.

Fig. 416.—Hyperplasia of the root of the maxillary right second premolar associated with granuloma.

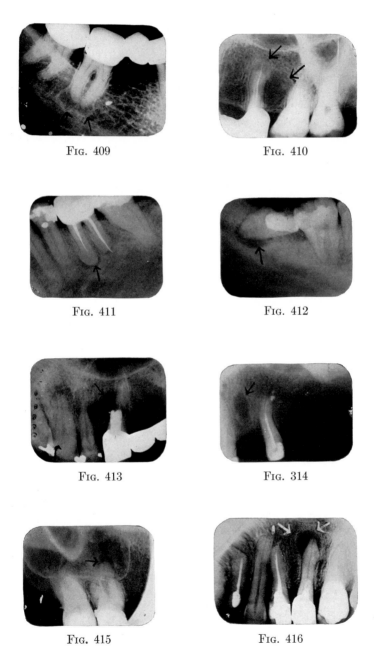

FIG. 409

FIG. 410

FIG. 411

FIG. 412

FIG. 413

FIG. 314

FIG. 415

FIG. 416

Figs. 417 to 424.—**Chronic Rarefying Osteitis With Granulation Tissue.**

Figs. 417, 418 and 419.—Granuloma commonly found in the apical region of pulpless teeth.

Fig. 420.—Granuloma of the maxillary right second incisor and first premolar. The radiolucent areas produced by the granuloma have extended until they are one. It does not involve the canine, which is a vital tooth, and the apical region of the canine may be observed to extend above the radiolucent area.

Fig. 421.—Absorption of the apical third of the maxillary left second incisor associated with granuloma.

Fig. 422.—Horizontal absorption of the alveolar process with a granuloma in the apical region of the right second incisor.

Fig. 423.—Granuloma involving the apical and middle third of the root of the lower left first premolar.

Fig. 424.—Extensive granuloma involving both roots of the mandibular left first molar, showing the typical appearance of the margin of the granuloma.

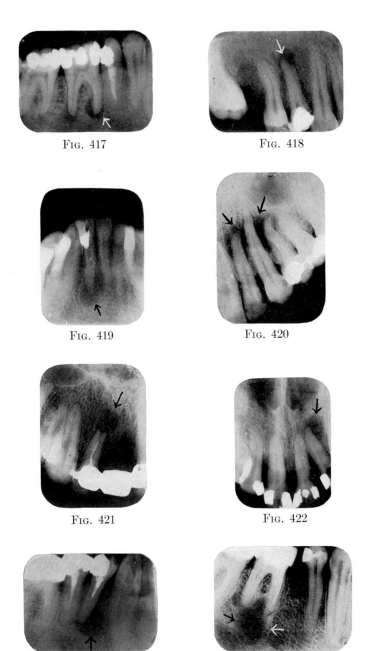

FIG. 417

FIG. 418

FIG. 419

FIG. 420

FIG. 421

FIG. 422

FIG. 423

FIG. 424

Figs. 425 to 432.—**Chronic Rarefying Osteitis With Granulation Tissue.**

Fig. 425.—The radiolucent area over the lingual root of the first molar gives the root the appearance of absorption. But the area is a granuloma on the mesial buccal root.

Fig. 426.—When taken at a different angle the tip of the lingual root becomes much longer, excluding any indication of absorption of the root.

Figs. 427 and 428.—Granuloma involving the second premolar and the first and second molars. This illustration is interesting in that the mandibular second premolar shows two roots.

Fig. 429.—Granuloma involving the maxillary left second incisor and the canine, the radiolucent areas extending upward to the floor of the nose.

Fig. 430.—Granuloma formed on the residual root under a restoration.

Fig. 431.—Granuloma in the apical region of the mandibular left first molar. The tooth has the clinical appearance of being healthy, but caries under the filling has evidently devitalized the tooth to cause the existing condition.

Fig. 432.—Granuloma in the apical region of the second premolar superimposed over the maxillary sinus.

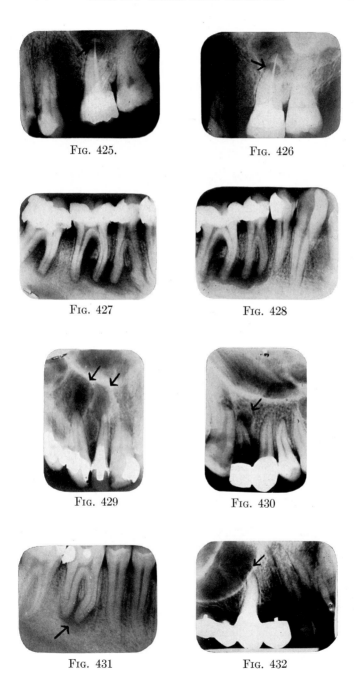

FIG. 425.

FIG. 426

FIG. 427

FIG. 428

FIG. 429

FIG. 430

FIG. 431

FIG. 432

These areas of bone rarefaction and destruction vary greatly in size. The bone absorption is usually accompanied by a slow detachment and destruction of the alveolo-dental periosteum covering the cementum of the root end, thus depriving the root end of its blood supply and converting it into a necrotic foreign body.

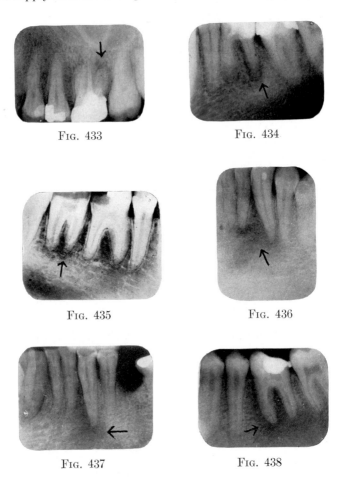

FIG. 433   FIG. 434

FIG. 435   FIG. 436

FIG. 437   FIG. 438

FIGS. 433 to 438.—**Chronic Rarefying Osteitis With Suppuration.**

Illustrations show the typical appearance of the bone when a suppurative condition is present. The area is diffuse and it is impossible definitely to locate the periphery of the area. The infection passes into the normal bone to produce this diffused margin, having no limiting membrane as found in indications of granuloma.

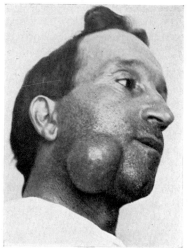

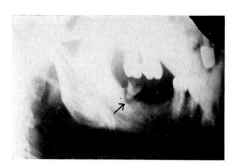

FIG. 440

FIG. 439

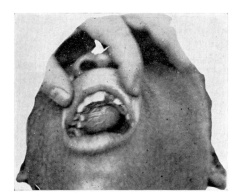

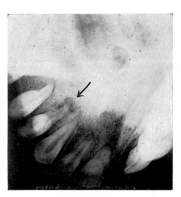

FIG. 441 FIG. 442

FIGS. 439 to 442.—**Rarefying Osteitis With Suppuration.**

FIG. 439.—Case of swelling on the outside of the face. Inflated part filled with pus, caused by the condition seen in the roentgenogram Fig. 440.

FIG. 440.—Showing a residual root of the mandibular third molar. Infection from this root, following the line of least resistance, has passed through the outer alveolar plate and adjoining tissues.

FIG. 441.—Swelling on the palate the size of a walnut filled with pus, its origin being the condition appearing in the roentgenogram Fig. 442.

FIG. 442.—A suppurative condition involving the apical region of the maxillary right first premolar.

Important from the clinical standpoint is that the contents of the spaces, including bacteria and their products, produced by periapical bone absorption are directly connected with the general circulation through the blood-vessels and lymphatics in the walls of the cavities, and running in all directions through the granulation tissue; and while the outer layers of the granulation tissue may be denser and more fibrous than its inner portion, tending to prevent local spread of infection there is no positive limiting membrane in the sense of preventing its contents from entering the general circulation and being deposited in distant structures of the body.

CHRONIC RAREFYING OSTEITIS WITH SUPPURATION.

Etiology.—The access of streptococci to the apical alveolo-dental periosteum usually causes a typical inflammatory reaction. The streptococcus is of the hemolytic type—of high virulence. The suppurative condition is grafted upon a chronic rarefying osteitis. The resistance of the patient is usually low.

Symptoms.—Swelling associated with pain; teeth at first seem to be raised in their sockets, and later become loose.

Roentgenographic Abnormalities.—The roentgenogram presents a blurred area of somewhat lessened density compared with the surrounding bone; presents irregular and ill-defined margins, into which the roughened tooth apex projects. The more active the suppurative process, the more irregular and ill-defined will be the margins of the lesion in the roentgenogram. The infection in this type is to be regarded as more active than in the forms of rarefying osteitis with granulation tissue. (Figs. 433 to 446, pages 286 to 289.)

Acute Exacerbation of a Chronic Rarefying Osteitis With Granulation Tissue.—An acute dento-alveolar abscess develops from a chronic rarefying osteitis with granulation tissue, with all the clinical symptoms of an acute inflammatory condition. The connective-tissue elements in the granulation tissue break down, forming an abscess cavity filled with pus. (Figs. 443 to 446.)

Among the connective-tissue elements of the inflammatory granulation tissue developing as a result of infection about the root apex are frequently found masses of squamous epithelial cells. Similar cells are present normally in the alveolo-dental periosteum, where they are known as the paradental epithelial cell-rests of Malassez.

(Fig. 447.) These epithelial cells are believed to be the remains of the outer cells of the enamel organ, which originally passed down and formed the outer wall of the sac in which the cementum of the

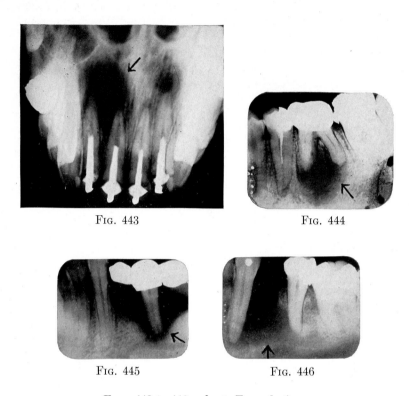

FIG. 443

FIG. 444

FIG. 445

FIG. 446

FIGS. 443 to 446.—**Acute Exacerbation.**

FIG. 443.—An acute suppurative condition grafted upon an old chronic rarefying osteitis.

FIG. 444.—Acute condition grafted upon an old chronic rarefying osteitis.

FIG. 445.—An acute suppurative condition associated with a vertical absorption of the alveolar process.

FIG. 446.—An acute suppurative area, following the extraction of the first premolar.

root was formed. (Fig. 448.) Proliferation of these epithelial cells found among the granulation tissue is stimulated by the chronic inflammatory process. The mass of epithelium then breaks down in the center, forming a cavity containing fluid. This cyst

19

cavity gradually enlarges because of the continued pressure of the proliferating epithelial cells, causing atrophy of the central epithelial cells. Due to this continued pressure, the surrounding granulation tissue is forced to the periphery of the enlarging bone cavity; and, eventually, the walls of the cyst consist of a dense fibrous capsule lined with a few layers of epithelial cells. The cyst fluid is usually clear, usually sterile; but infection of the cyst wall frequently

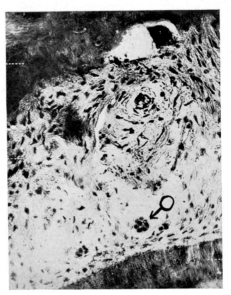

Fig. 447.—Arrow pointing to the epithelial cell-rests of Malassez, which are found normally in the alveolo-dental periosteum and is the source from whence the epithelium of a cyst is derived. (Courtesy of Dr. Hopewell-Smith.)

converts the cystic content into pus. Dental root cysts vary considerably in size. In the maxilla, they may push up the floor of the maxillary sinus or of the nasal fossa, but rarely do they actually open into these cavities. Recently a number of these cysts have been reported closely associated with carcinoma, and with the suggestion that they may have degenerated into carcinoma.

Usually the dental root cyst is sterile, its greatest evil being its destruction of the bone by pressure, a destruction sometimes so great as to cause a pathological fracture. Such cysts should be recognized and removed in their incipience. They should never be treated through a root canal by medication, but must be removed surgically, as the entire epithelial wall must be removed to prevent recurrence. Cysts do often become infected after the extraction of teeth by reason of the invasion of bacteria from the oral cavity.

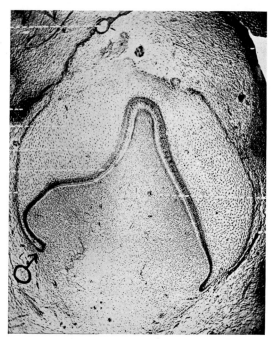

Fig. 448.—Arrow pointing to the outer and inner layer of epithelium of the enamel organ, which join together and form the epithelial sheath of Hertwig. (Courtesy of Dr. Hopewell-Smith.)

CHRONIC RAREFYING OSTEITIS WITH CYST FORMATION

Etiology.—Stimulation to activity and rapid growth of the epithelial "rests of Malassez," found in the alveolo-dental periosteum. Cut off from their blood supply, the central epithelial cells die, degenerate and liquefy, and a cyst results. This theory has been fully investigated and described by J. G. Turner.[1]

Symptoms.—A slow progressive swelling, unaccompanied by pain. Inflammation and suppuration may occur as a secondary change, and degeneration into carcinoma is not beyond possibility.

Roentgenographic Abnormalities.—This stage succeeds that of rarefying osteitis with granulation tissue. The cavity in the bone is

[1] Journal British Dental Association, 1898.

Figs. 449 to 456.—Chronic Rarefying Osteitis With Cyst Formation.

Fig. 449.—Residual cyst in the region of the maxillary left second incisor. Note the well-defined margins of the area. This condition was found in a man seventy years of age.

Fig. 450.—Cyst in the apical region of an undeveloped maxillary left first incisor.

Fig. 451.—Cyst in the apical region of the maxillary right and left first incisors. Both teeth are apparently vital. However, note the thickening of the alveolo-dental periosteum in the apical region of the right first incisor, a tooth that was partially vital.

Fig. 452.—Large cyst in the anterior portion of the palate involving the four maxillary incisors. The right and left first incisors have been fractured, the apical thirds of both teeth noticeably lying in the cyst cavity. The fracture was in all possibility due to trauma, though history unknown.

Fig. 453.—Residual cyst in the region of the maxillary left third molar. The lower wall of the cyst is broken, causing the cystic fluid to be continually poured into the mouth.

Fig. 454.—Residual cyst associated with the residual roots of the maxillary left first molar, the cyst extending into the maxillary sinus, but having no direct connection or communication with the sinus.

Fig. 455.—Infected cyst extending into the maxillary sinus over the right second premolar and first molar.

Fig. 456.—Cyst in the wall of the maxillary sinus over the right second premolar.

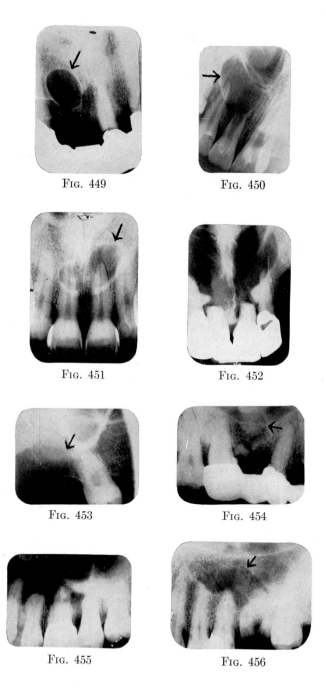

FIG. 449

FIG. 450

FIG. 451

FIG. 452

FIG. 453

FIG. 454

FIG. 455

FIG. 456

Figs. 457 to 462.—**Chronic Rarefying Osteitis With Cyst Formation.**

Fig. 457.—Residual cyst in the region of the mandibular right first molar.

Fig. 458.—An occlusal view of Fig. 457, showing the cyst and the amount of destruction of the outer and inner plates of the mandible.

Fig. 459.—Large cyst involving the maxillary right first premolar. Root-canal treatment was attempted, but failed. This cyst was successfully treated finally by surgical removal.

Fig. 460.—A recurrent cyst in the mandible. The original cyst was removed, but evidently some of the epithelial lining remained to result in having another cyst formed as here shown.

Fig. 461.—Patient complained of having a discharge from the region of the maxillary left first molar. The roentgenogram reveals a necrotic condition in that area, but does not show the cause. An occlusal film was then used for the same case with the result shown in Fig. 462.

Fig. 462.—Showing an infected cyst as a radiopaque area in the maxillary sinus, but having no direct connection with the sinus.

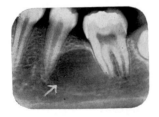

FIG. 457

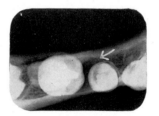

FIG. 458

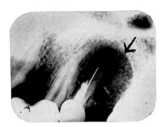

FIG. 459

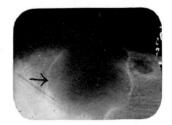

FIG. 460

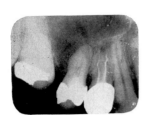

FIG. 461

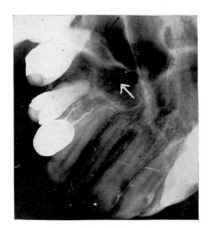

FIG. 462

filled with clear fluid and often with some soft tissue, together with a thin fibrous sac; and in the roentgenogram, therefore, the cyst appears as a very clearly defined radiolucent area involving the apices of one of more teeth. The margins are regular and very sharply defined, so that there is usually no difficulty in determining where the healthy bone ends. (Figs. 449 to 470, pages 293 to 298.)

The principal stages of chronic periapical disease giving rise to roentgenographic abnormalities may be summed up as follows:

1. Chronic proliferative alveolo-dental periostitis.
2. Chronic rarefying osteitis with granulation tissue.
3. Chronic rarefying osteitis with suppuration.
4. Chronic rarefying osteitis with cyst formation.

II. LESIONS INVOLVING THE INVESTING TISSUES OF THE TEETH.

For a detailed discussion of the etiology and pathology of chronic suppurative alveolo-dental periostitis, or pyorrhea alveolaris, the reader is urgently referred to the thoroughly excellent treatise in Dr. Herman Prinz's *Soft Structures of the Teeth and Their Treatment* (Part II), and to Prof. Arthur Hopewell-Smith's *Normal and Pathological Histology of the Mouth* (vol. 2). Only meagerly are such points as have a direct bearing upon roentgenographic findings alluded to in this present work.

Alveolo-dental periostitis may be caused by either a systemic or a local cause, and it is safe to say that a majority of the cases result from local causes. Various consititutional diseases that lower the vital resistance of the individual are predisposing factors. However, the disease always begins as a gingivitis due to some local irritation of the gum tissue about the gingival margin. Among these irritating factors may be mentioned: malocclusion, improper contact of teeth produced by faulty restorative operations, imperfect margins of crowns and fillings, lack of cleanliness—all of which will produce a local injury to the gum tissue and permit infection by the micro-organisms always present in the mouth.

At first, the lesion is confined to the gum tissue, producing a gingivitis, and registering no roentgenographic changes. Later the alveolo-dental periosteum is attacked, becoming thereby a chronic gingivo-alveolo-dental periostitis, the infection progressing slowly from the gum margin toward the apex of the tooth. In the roentgenogram this stage shows a thickening of the normal alveolo-dental periosteal radiolucent line. Very soon after involvement of

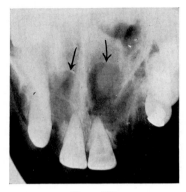

FIG. 463

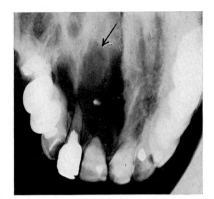

FIG. 464

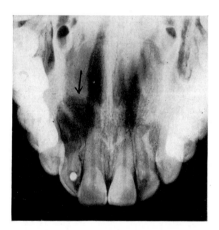

FIG. 465

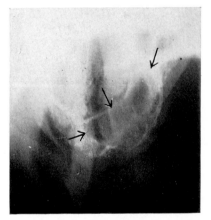

FIG. 466

FIGS. 463 to 466.—Chronic rarefying osteitis with cyst formation. Cysts may be unilateral or bilateral, may be small or large, are generally noninfectious but cause considerable damage due to their tendency continually to expand.

FIG. 463.—A bilateral cyst in the anterior region of the palate.

FIG. 464.—A unilateral cyst causing a considerable amount of destruction.

FIG. 465.—A cyst associated with an undeveloped maxillary left second incisor.

FIG. 466.—A large cyst in an edentulous mouth.

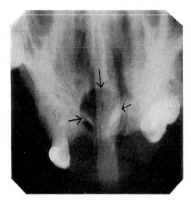

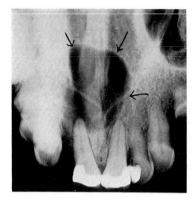

Fig. 467   Fig. 468

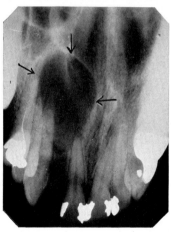

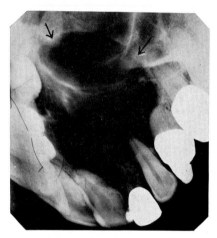

Fig. 469   Fig. 470

Figs. 467 to 470.—Rarefying osteitis with cyst. Chronic rarefying osteitis with cyst formation, illustrating how cysts continually destroy the bony structures. The proportions to which unattended cysts may develop are shown in the separate cases represented.

Fig. 467.—Small cyst in the median line in the anterior portion of the palate.

Fig. 468.—A cyst much larger than in Fig. 467.

Fig. 469.—A cyst slightly larger than in Fig. 468.

Fig. 470.—A cyst covering two-thirds of the palate.

the alveolo-dental periosteum, the bone itself becomes affected, this being first manifested in the roentgenogram by the absence of the apex of the bony septum between the teeth. And the bone surrounding the tooth may be progressively destroyed toward the apex of the tooth, and the entire bony support of the tooth lost.

Thus we would have an osteo-alveolo-dental periostitis, which disease may be classified into two types, the vertical and the horizontal. When the infection is localized around an individual tooth it is designated the vertical type (Figs. 476 to 479); but when a number of adjoining teeth are affected it is designated the horizontal type. (Figs. 480 to 485.)

Pyorrhea, that is, the pus itself, cannot be diagnosed from the roentgenogram. Only the effect of the disease on the alveolar process can be seen, this manifesting itself in an absorbing of the alveolar process. As there are other conditions which cause a similarly appearing absorption of the alveolar process, senile atrophy and occlusal trauma for example, it is inaccurate to diagnose the loss of the alveolar process as seen in the roentgnogram as pyorrhea. It should be interpreted as a vertical absorption of the alveolar process or a horizontal absorption of the alveolar process, as the case may be. The cause of the absorption must be diagnosed by a clinical examination.

The principal stages of chronic suppurative alveolo-dental periostitis as seen in the roentgenogram may be summed up as follows:

1. Gingivitis: no roentgenographic change.

2. Chronic gingivo-alveolo-dental periostitis: thickening of the normal alveolo-dental periosteal radiolucent line.

3. Osteo-alveolo-dental periostitis: the loss of bone shown by a lessening in density, which in advanced cases may completely surround the tooth.

Roentgenographic study of cases of chronic suppurative alveolo-dental periostitis is of highest importance in order to determine the extent of bone destruction so that the proper course of treatment may be decided.

PERIOSTEAL ABSCESS.

Etiology.—Most cases of periosteal abscesses are caused by infection gaining access to the alveolo-dental periosteum through the gingival margin, and setting up a chronic inflammatory process that later becomes a suppurative condition. It is generally found in the region of the maxillary incisors, and in the bifurcations of multi-rooted teeth.

Symptoms.—The conditions shown in a swelling, usually accompanied by considerable pain.

Roentgenographic Findings.—A radiolucent area in the affected region will appear on the negative.

A periosteal abscess is one of the most difficult types of infection to distinguish, and, therefore, to interpret, in a roentgenogram. Clinically, the teeth may respond to the electric test for vitality

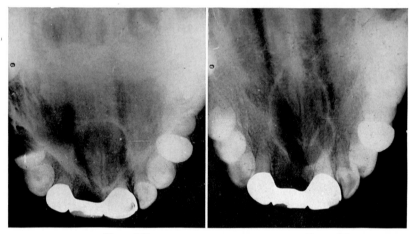

Fig. 471   Fig. 472

Figs. 471 and 472.—A residual cyst in the medial line, probably the result of infection remaining after the first incisor was extracted.

Fig. 471.—Rays directed perpendicular, showing probably the true form of the cyst while in Fig. 472 the area has become elongated due to angulation.

Legends for Figs. 473, 474, and 475.

Figs. 473, 473, and 475.—A skull showing the effects of a large dental root cyst.

Fig. 473.—Shows the outer alveolar plate to be broken down over the left first incisor and second premolar.

Fig. 474.—A palatal view; shows the destruction taken place and its extension into the nose.

Fig. 475.—Shows the destruction on the outer plate of the alveolus with the breaking down of the bone over the first premolar and depicts the roots of the teeth communicating with the area. This specimen is the property of Dr. Oscar V. Batson.

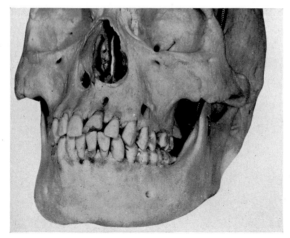

Fig. 473

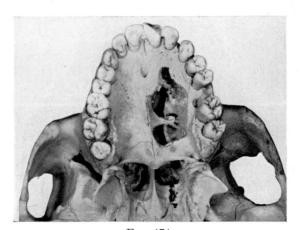

Fig. 474

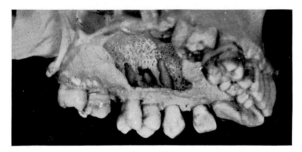

Fig. 475

because the pulp may be unaffected. But cases arise in non-vital teeth, as we find these abscesses exist where root-canal fillings are present. (Fig. 486.)

CONDENSING OSTEITIS.

After eradication of infection in a periapical bone area, new bone is usually formed, filling in the space after several months. The bone cells of the surrounding alveolar process deposit lime salts,

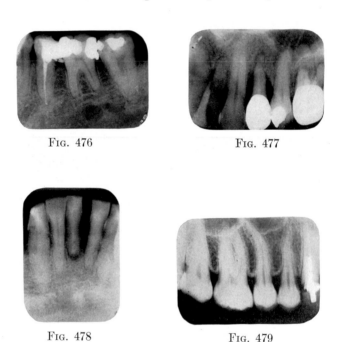

Fig. 476   Fig. 477

Fig. 478   Fig. 479

FIGS. 476 to 479.—Vertical Absorption of the Alveolar Process.

FIG. 476.—Vertical absorption caused by over-hanging fillings.
FIG. 477.—Vertical absorption caused by ill-fitting crown.
FIG. 478.—Vertical absorption caused by improper contact of the teeth.
GIG. 479.—Vertical absorption between the maxillary canine and first premolar due to very poor restoration.

the density gradually increasing until normal bone is the result. Occasionally this new bone is denser than normal, due to excessive deposit of lime salts, and is shown in the roentgenogram as a radi-

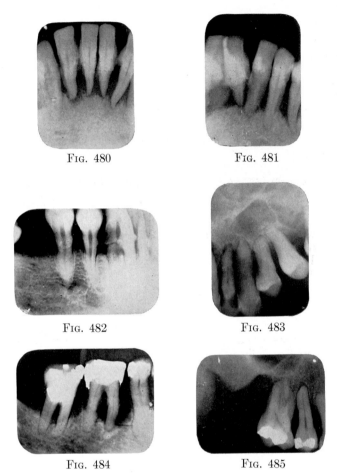

Fig. 480   Fig. 481

Fig. 482   Fig. 483

Fig. 484   Fig. 485

FIGS. 480 to 485.—Horizontal absorption of the alveolar process, illustrating various degrees of horizontal absorption of the alveolar process. Fig. 480 shows large amounts of calculus attached to the teeth.

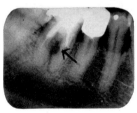

FIG. 486.—An alveolo-dental periosteal abscess in the bifurcation of the roots of the first molar.

Figs. 487 to 495.—**Condensing Osteitis.**

Fig. 487.—Absorption of the mesial root of the mandibular first molar with a condensing osteitis taking the place of the root.

Fig. 488.—Same as Fig. 487, but with the filling removed and both tested for vitality. Tooth responded to the test, the nerve supply coming from the distal root.

Fig. 489.—Same case as Fig. 487, but with the tooth removed. Under an impression of there being a part of the root remaining, the operator then tried unsuccessfully to remove the condensed bone with an elevator.

Fig. 490—Absorption of the second premolar associated with a condensing osteitis.

Fig. 491.—Right and left side of the same mouth. On the right side there are two areas of condensing osteitis in the region of the mandibular first molar, while on the left side there is a large area of condensing osteitis on the distal root of the first molar which is partly absorbed.

Fig. 492.—Condensing osteitis in the apical region of the mandibular right first molar, which tooth was vital.

Fig. 493.—Condensing osteitis of the mandible in the region of the mandibular first molar, which has been extracted.

Fig. 494.—Condensing osteitis anterior to the mesial root of the mandibular first molar; the condensing osteitis in this case is probably due to a trauma.

Fig. 495.—Condensing osteitis in the apical region of the mandibular first molar; in this particular case the condensing osteitis in all probability was due to trauma.

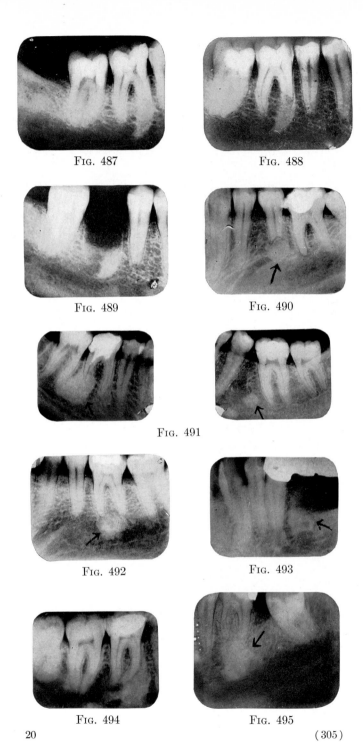

FIG. 487

FIG. 488

FIG. 489

FIG. 490

FIG. 491

FIG. 492

FIG. 493

FIG. 494

FIG. 495

opaque area. (Figs. 487 to 495.) This dense bone may, in isolated cases, contribute a pressure on peripheral nerve endings to cause neuralgia.

But there are cases where a condition of root absorption has been followed by a natural generation of new bone, without there having been any treatment for the removal of the infection. (Figs. 525 and 526.)

An Nature has similarly supplied new and denser bone structure to compensate for irregular inclination of teeth that are often found in the mandibular molar region. (Figs. 494, 620 and 622.) Chronic inflammations do not always lead to bone destruction. Low-grade irritations of long standing, instead of destroying bone, sometimes cause a hypertrophy in a circumscribed area.

The pliability of the alveolar process lends itself easily to the constantly protecting ends of Nature in its course of contributing and depositing an increasing supply of bony structure for the support of over-burdened teeth. Often, because of extractions or other factors, the burden that should be borne by two or several teeth is imposed upon one. Figs. 620 to 622 show the reconstruction of bone to support teeth out of their normal axial lines and called upon to perform an abnormally excessive duty. The medullary spaces of cancellated bone are never of any definite size or shape, and in the roentgenogram appear as large radiolucent areas (Fig. 624), which may be mistaken for some pathological process.

Sometimes, due to the absorption process that may take place in the root of a tooth, there is gradually deposited new bone that has practically the normal density of the surrounding process. (Figs. 621 and 626.) At other times, however, the bone so deposited in the region of absorbed roots or in areas formerly occupied by some pathological process may be in excess of the normal amount and density. (Figs. 487, 488 and 489.) Formerly called "bone whorls," now we speak of these areas as indicating "condensing osteitis."

PATHOLOGICAL CONDITIONS OF THE DENTINE AS SEEN IN THE ROENTGENOGRAM.

1. **Adventitious Dentine.**—"Tissue of a pathological nature which has been added, in the course of dental caries, and in erosion, to the primary or first formed dentine." (Hopewell-Smith.)

Inflammation of the pulp produces a stimulation of the peripheral cells of the pulp, which lays down a new form of dentine. This condition appears in the roentgenogram as a constriction of the normal radiolucent pulp chamber, the constriction being due to the addition of the new dentine. Adventitious dentine is radiopaque,

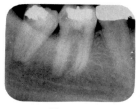 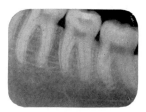

Fig. 496   Fig. 497

Figs. 496 and 497.—Adventitious dentine. Note the loss of the horns of the pulp chamber by the addition of new dentine.

and generally seen in the roof of the pulp chamber, either one or sometimes both horns of the pulp chamber being obliterated. (Figs. 496 and 497.)

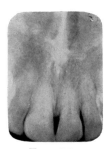 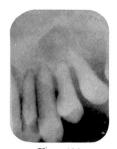

Fig. 498   Fig. 499

Figs. 498 and 499.—Senile dentine. Note the obliteration of the pulp chambers and the root canals.

2. **Senile Dentine.**—The dentine of old age may be attributed to a diminished supply of nutrition causing trophic changes, first in the pulp tissue and, second, in the hard tissues. In the roentgenogram the pulp shows very small and the root canals are practically obliterated. (Figs. 498 and 499.)

3. **Calcareous Degeneration of the Pulp.**—The degenerations are divided into two classes: (*a*) Where the new material is unattached to the walls of the pulp cavity; and (*b*) where it is attached.

(*a*) Lime-salt deposits which are unattached to the walls of pulp take the form of nodules or rods. Pulp nodules originate near the center of the pulp, close to the vascular system. They may appear in all types of teeth, and at practically all ages. The roengenogram reveals them as radiopaque areas within the radiolucent pulp. (Figs. 500 and 501.)

(*b*) Lime-salt deposits or attached deposits of dentine are seen in the cervical or coronal portions of the pulp. They generally occur where there have been pathological changes of the dentine.

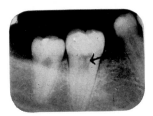 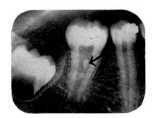

| Fig. 500 | Fig. 501 |

Fig. 500.—Pulp nodules in the mandibular left second molar.

Fig. 501.—Dentine not fully developed separating the mesial and distal canals of a single-rooted mandibular molar.

Partial calcification of the pulp generally occurs in adults. Long rods of calcific material run longitudinally through the pulp, and are seen in the roentgenogram as long, spindle-shaped radiopaque areas extending throughout the entire length of the pulp. (Fig. 502.)

Complete calcification of the pulp occurs in adults and in some instances in younger persons where the tooth has received a traumatic injury. The long rods of calcific material fuse and ultimately obliterate all traces of the pulp. This condition appears in the roentgenogram as a radiopaque area which has entirely obliterated the normal radiolucent area of the root canal and pulp chamber. (Fig. 503.)

Dilaceration.—Malformation of the teeth, in which the hard structures are derived from the axial straight line in such a way as to form an angle with it. It may be caused by a blow or by some

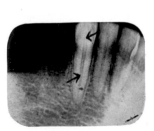 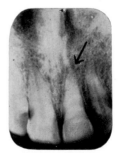

Fig. 502   Fig. 503

Fig. 502.—Partial calcification of the pulp, showing the entire pulp undergoing a degenerative change.

Fig. 503.—Complete calcification of the pulp in the maxillary right first incisor, the entire pulp chamber having been obliterated.

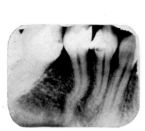 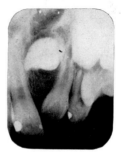

Fig. 504   Fig. 505

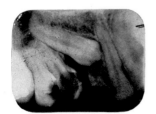 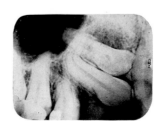

Fig. 506   Fig. 507

Figs. 504 to 507.—**Dilaceration.**

Fig. 504.—Dilacertion of the mandibular left second premolar.

Fig. 505.—Dilaceration of the maxillary right first incisor.

Fig. 506.—Dilaceration of an impacted maxillary left canine.

Fig. 507.—Impacted maxillary second incisor and canine associated with a dilaceration of the maxillary canine.

abnormal condition preventing its normal eruption, the root developing and forming in the line of least resistance. In the roentgenogram the teeth may be seen in the process of development deviating
out of the axial straight line. Teeth which have fully developed
show roots distorted. (Figs. 504 to 507.)

Gemination.—The union of two or more teeth is divided into two
classes—"true" and "false."

True gemination is the term applied to those teeth which are
joined together during developmental periods, and in the roentgenogram show the existence of a common pulp chamber (Figs. 508,
509 and 510) and a union of the enamel and the dentine.

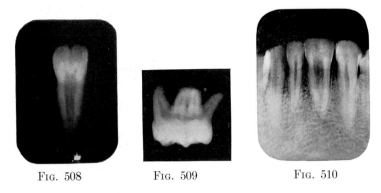

| Fig. 508 | Fig. 509 | Fig. 510 |

Figs. 508 to 510.—**True Gemination.**

Fig. 508.—True gemination of the mandibular incisors.
Fig. 509.—True gemination of the maxillary molars. There is one
common pulp chamber in each case.
Fig. 510.—Showing a true gemination of the right mandibular first and
second incisors, the two teeth having a common pulp chamber and canal.

False gemination is the result of a productive periostitis, which
causes the osteoblasts of the root membrane to lay down an overgrowth of cementum. In the roentgenogram, therefore, the affected
teeth show two distinct pulp chambers and a union of the dentine
only. (Figs. 511 to 514.)

Diphyodontic gemination is that condition in which a deciduous
tooth may become firmly united to a member of the permanent
series. (Figs. 515 to 517.)

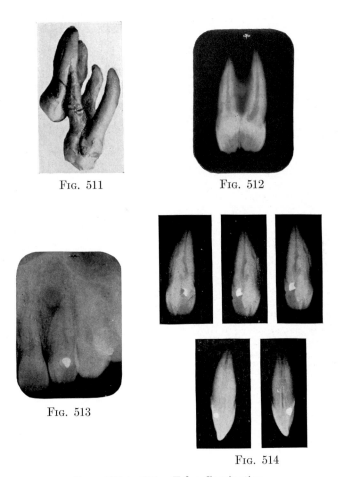

Fig. 511   Fig. 512

Fig. 513

Fig. 514

Figs. 511 to 514.—**False Gemination.**

Fig. 511.—Two maxillary molars joined by false gemination.

Fig. 512.—False gemination of the canine and second incisor. There are two distinct pulp chambers, this type of gemination occurring after the tooth is developed.

Fig. 513.—False gemination between the right first incisor and a supernumerary tooth. There is a rarefied area in the apical region. The tooth was opened, and the operator found it to be very vital. Not interpreting condition properly, as it should have been, as a false gemination that the roentgenogram indicates, the tooth was then extracted.

Fig. 514.—Same case as Fig. 513 after extraction. Roentgenograms of the tooth show two distinct pulp chambers.

ABSORPTION OF THE TEETH.

Absorption is the removal or destruction of dentine and cementum. In deciduous teeth it is a physiological process. But in permanent teeth it is part of a pathological process.

It is with the permanent teeth, with the pathological causation of absorption, that the dentist meets problems; for any assumptions as to explanations of the cause of absorption have only theories of diverging reasoning to support them. It is generally conceded to be the result of some action of the multi-nucleated giant cells or to the presence of absorption leukocytes or phagocytes brought into contact with the teeth as through some inflammatory condition.

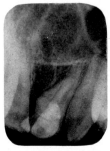 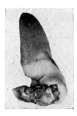 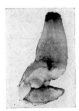

FIG. 515   FIG. 516   FIG. 517

FIGS. 515 to 517.—**Diphyodontic Gemination.**

FIG. 515.—Roentgenogram of the maxillary right first incisor, showing a diphyodontic gemination.
FIGS. 516 and 517.—Photographs of the same after extraction.

Hopewell-Smith suggests that "Multi-nucleated giant cells have to be regarded as aggregations of protoplasm derived from cells that have been exhausted in giving off a digestive ferment . . . which is credited with the action of absorption." Absorption comprehends the physiological and pathological destruction of the cementum and dentine of the teeth, to which he has applied the terms:

Osteolysis—a dissolution of the bone.

Odontolysis—a dissolution of the tooth structures.

The process of osteolysis is brought about during a condition which we may call subacute inflammatory, wherein slow-moving cells appear—mononuclear leukocytes and plasma cells. The latter are credited by Maximow with liberating a digestive ferment possibly acid in nature. The liberated ferments of these plasma cells dissolve the bone or tooth structure forming Howship's lacuna; in doing so their function becomes exhausted and they die. Finally, their protoplasm coalesces and forms with the débris of the osteolyzed structure large aggregations which have hitherto been called giant cells. They appear as large multinucleated cells in which, however, location of nuclei is atypical. The outline of the so-called giant cells, and the fact that we see these aggregations splitting up or coalescing, suggests the absence of individuality of these so-called giant cells. It seems now the task of the mononuclear leukocytes to act as scavengers and pick up the débris of structures and cells to carry them off in the well-known way.

Osteolysis may be divided into three stages:

1. Abstraction of the lime salts.
2. Bone undergoes a change into an osteoid structure.
3. Osteoid structure undergoes further change into a fibrous structure.

Between the first and third stages a condition exists known as osteoporosis or spongy bone, characterized by an increase in size of the Haversian canals and medullary spaces. When fibrous structure disappears the bone is completely dissolved and osteolysis or odontolysis has taken place.

The direction the absorption process takes in a tooth must be accurately determined, for there are two distinct trend directions. In the first type are those cases where absorption begins from the external surface or cementum side, often easily ascribable to some local condition—an infection, perhaps, or pressure from other teeth. In the second type are cases where absorption begins from the interior or pulpal part of the tooth.

External Absorption.—External absorption is very common, occurring generally in non-vital teeth, and starting in the apical region and continuing until the entire tooth may be absorbed. (Figs. 518 to 531.)

It is a very destructive process from its incipiency, though slow and usually painless. But when the apex of the tooth presents a "needle point" absorption (Fig. 524), any movement of the tooth may cause considerable discomfort and become positively painful. And also, where absorption of a vital tooth is induced by an impaction giving rise to an acute inflammation of the alveolo-dental periosteum associated with suppuration, great pain may be experienced.

Figs. 518 to 525.—**Absorption (External).**

Fig. 518.—Roots of a deciduous molar absorbed; the premolar is absent.

Fig. 519.—Deciduous molar with roots not fully absorbed; the premolar being absent.

Fig. 520.—Absorption of the distal root of the mandibular left second molar.

Fig. 521.—External absorption of the first molar.

Fig. 522.—Absorption of the root supporting a bridge.

Fig. 523.—Practically the entire root of the mandibular premolar supporting the bridge has been absorbed.

Fig. 524.—Needle-point absorption of the mandibular left second incisor.

Fig. 525.—Absorption of the lingual root of the first molar.

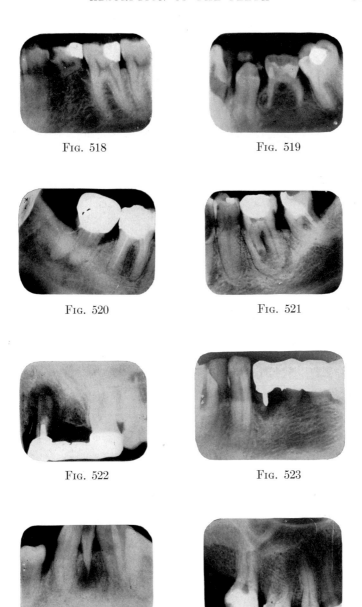

FIG. 518

FIG. 519

FIG. 520

FIG. 521

FIG. 522

FIG. 523

FIG. 524

FIG. 525

Figs. 526 to 534.—**Absorption (External).**

Fig. 526.—Absorption of the root of a replanted maxillary right first incisor.

Fig. 527.—Absorption of the apical and middle third of the root of the maxillary left first incisor.

Fig. 528.—Absorption of the apical third of the maxillary left first incisor, the tooth being associated with a cyst.

Fig. 529.—Irregular absorption of the maxillary left first incisor. The second incisor is also affected.

Fig. 530.—Practically a complete absorption of the root of the maxillary left first incisor. It has been supporting a Richmond crown that is now being held in place by the adjoining teeth and the alveolar process.

Fig. 531.—Absorption of the maxillary first incisor, showing a condition of absorption not as far advanced as Fig. 530.

Fig. 532.—Absorption beginning from the pulpal side of the middle third of the maxillary right second incisor. This condition continues until the entire tooth is divided.

Fig. 533.—Absorption of the middle third of the maxillary right second incisor. This case is further advanced than Fig. 532.

Fig. 534.—The absorption process in a more advanced state; the right second incisor has been fully divided. The tooth was removed and appears in Fig. 535.

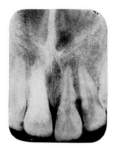

FIG 526

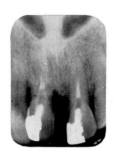

FIG. 527

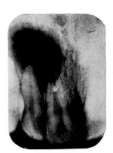

FIG. 528

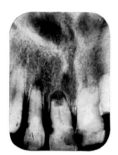

FIG. 529

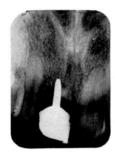

FIG. 530

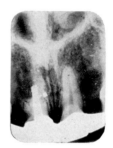

FIG. 531

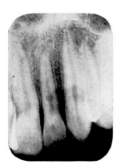

FIG. 532

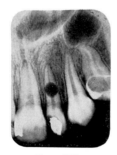

FIG. 533

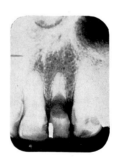

FIG. 534

Figs. 535 to 544.—**Absorption (Internal).**

Fig. 535.—Tooth seen in Fig. 534 photographed after extraction to show the similarity to the absorption seen in deciduous teeth.

Fig. 536.—Absorption of the middle third of the maxillary right first incisor.

Fig. 537.—Absorption of the middle third of the maxillary left second incisor.

Figs. 538 and 539.—Two views of the maxillary left second incisor, showing an absorption of the middle third of the root.

Figs. 540, 541 and 542.—Three photographic views of the tooth seen in Figs 538 and 539 after extraction, the lateral views showing a cavity in the middle third of the root Fig. 542.

Figs. 543 and 544.—Roentgenograms of the root of the tooth in Figs. 538 and 539 after extraction, illustrating the loss of tooth structure internally.

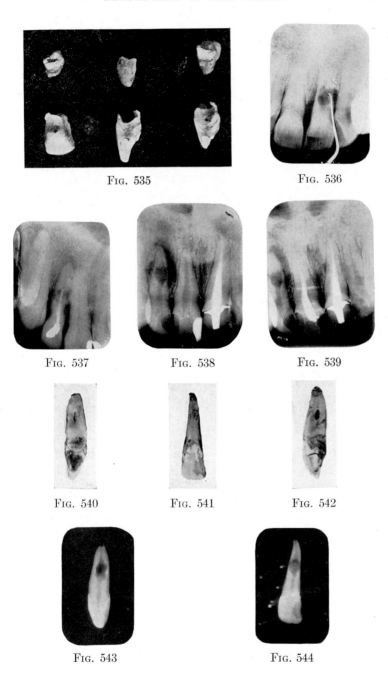

FIG. 535

FIG. 536

FIG. 537

FIG. 538

FIG. 539

FIG. 540

FIG. 541

FIG. 542

FIG. 543

FIG. 544

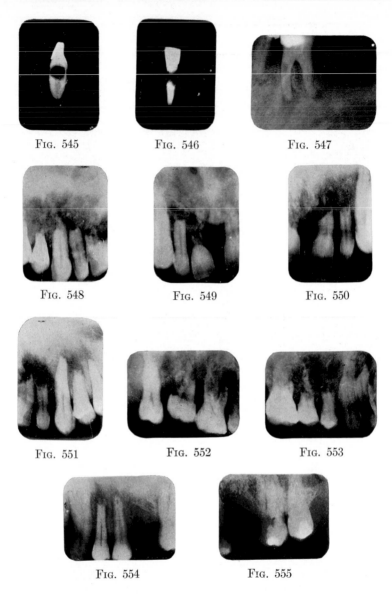

FIG. 545   FIG. 546   FIG. 547

FIG. 548   FIG. 549   FIG. 550

FIG. 551   FIG. 552   FIG. 553

FIG. 554   FIG. 555

FIGS. 545 to 555.—**Absorption (Internal).**

FIGS. 545 and 546.—Roentgenogram of the mandibular incisor after extraction, illustrating the internal absorption process.

FIG. 547.—Absorption of the middle third of the mesial root of the mandibular right first molar.

FIGS. 548 to 555.—Absorption affecting all the teeth of the maxilla, associated with an absorption of the alveolar process.

(320)

Internal Absorption.—Internal absorption has been extremely baffling to the pathologist. W. D. Miller, whose thorough research to determine the probable cause of the condition was reported in the *Dental Cosmos*, 1901, referred to it as "pink spot," because a pink spot showed in all teeth he has seen so affected.

Since then a long line of eminent pathologists has pursued the investigation searchingly. Mummery[1] reports finding a number of cases in which the "pink spot" had occurred near the gingival line and extensive absorption in their interiors, and says: "In pink-spot cases the inflammatory action is very chronic in nature. . . Suppuration plays no part in the process, but the irritant, whatever it may be, gives rise to a chronic inflammatory reaction leading to

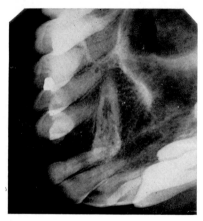

Fig. 556.—Absorption of a completely impacted maxillary left canine.

a localized breaking-down of portions of the pulp and their substitution by granulation tissue. . . It is peculiar that the condition seldom gives rise to pain and that the tooth is not sore to the touch."

Later, however, in the same journal of July, 1926, he reports a number of cases where the "pink spot" is wholly absent, and as more accurately describing the chief characteristics of the condition, he suggests the term "chronic perforating hyperplasia of the pulp."

In the roentgenogram it appear first as a small enlargement of the pulp cavity in a localized area (Fig. 532); but as the condition continues, the pathological process enlarges until the entire tooth may be divided. (Figs. 532 to 556.)

[1] Pink Spots on Teeth, British Dental Journal, April, 1920.

HYPERPLASIA OF THE CEMENTUM.

A thickening of the cementum due to an inflammatory reaction. It is a pathological overgrowth of the cementum,, and shows in the roentgenogram as an increase in the size of the apical portion of the root. It is radiopaque. (Figs. 557 to 562.)

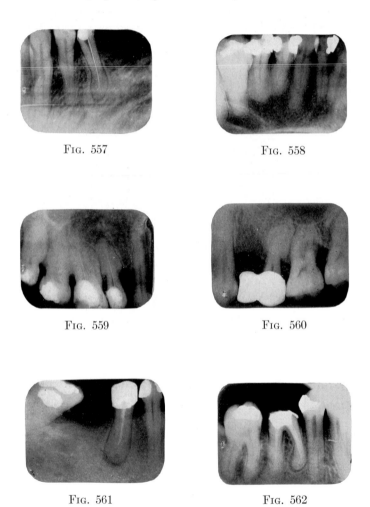

FIG. 557   FIG. 558

FIG. 559   FIG. 560

FIG. 561   FIG. 562

FIGS. 557 to 562.—Various types of hyperplasia of the cementum.

SIALOLITHS AND TONSILLITHS.

Sialoliths or salivary concretions found in the salivary ducts or glands are most commonly found in Wharton's duct or the submaxillary gland. They generally cause pain and swelling and

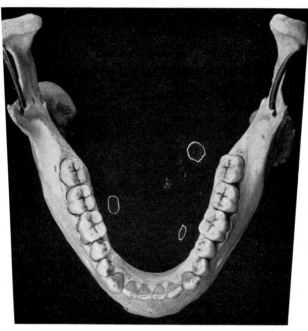

FIG. 563.—Various areas wherein salivary calculi are to be found in the floor of the mouth.

appear in the roentgenogram as a radiopaque area. They vary greatly in size, shape, and numbers. (Figs. 563 to 572.) Tonsilliths are the less common. They are salivary concretions found in the crypts of the tonsil, appearing radiopaque in the roentgenogram. (Figs. 570 and 572.)

Figs. 564 to 569.—**Salivary Calculi.**

Fig. 564.—Salivary calculus in the anterior portion of Wharton's duct.

Fig. 565.—Salivary calculus in the posterior portion of Wharton's duct, of which a roentgenogram was made after removal (Fig. 566).

Fig. 567.—Two salivary calculi found in Wharton's duct, one in the anterior portion, the other in the posterior portion.

Fig. 568.—Two salivary calculi found in the anterior portion of the floor of the mouth.

Fig. 569.—Salivary calculi found throughout the entire length of the Wharton duct.

Fig. 570.—Multilocular cyst in the region of the mandibular right canine; with a stone in the posterior portion of Wharton's duct.

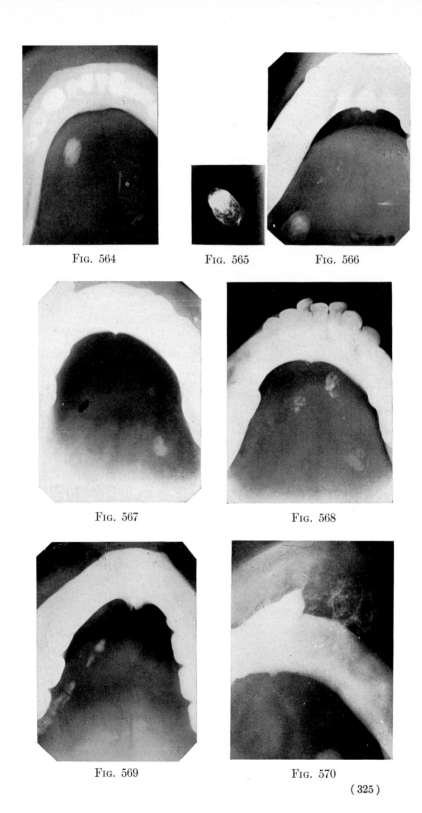

Fig. 564   Fig. 565   Fig. 566

Fig. 567   Fig. 568

Fig. 569   Fig. 570

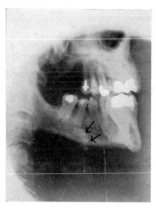

FIG. 571.—Arrows pointing to a radiopaque mass in the region of the second premolar. The mass is divided into two portions and extends below the lower border of the mandible. It indicates, therefore, that it is improbable that the radiopaque mass is attached to or is a part of the mandible. Notice the angle at which the roentgenogram was taken: the vertebra of the neck being superimposed over the ascending ramus denotes the rays to have been projected anteriorly, causing any substance or pathological condition found in the third molar region or in the area posterior to the ramus of the side nearest the tube to be projected or superimposed over the opposite side of the jaw in the region of the molar or premolar teeth. Thus this radiopaque mass may be interpreted as possibly a tonsillith or a salivary concretion found in the crypt of the tonsil. But the superimposition of the vertebra, over the ramus indicates the inaccurate angulation, and the roentgenogram should be taken properly as was done in Fig. 572.

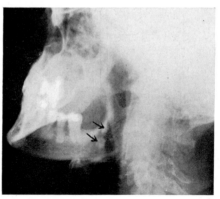

FIG. 572.—Arrows pointing to the tonsilliths found in Fig. 571, except that they are now back in the region where they approximately belong. The head is in the proper position and the angulation of the rays correct, allowing reproducing shadows of the mandible with the least amount of superimposing and distorting.

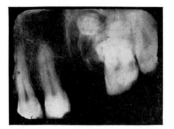

FIG. 573

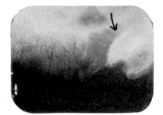   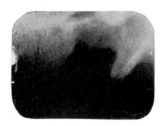

FIG. 574   FIG. 575

FIGS. 573 to 575.—**Parotid Calculi.**

FIG. 573.—Calculi found in the parotid gland several years after an injury. A condition such as this must undergo strict clinical examination, otherwise one might operate needlessly.

FIG. 574.—Arrow pointing to a piece of cotton covered with calculus and lying in the floor of the maxillary sinus. The cotton had been used in the socket of the first molar after extraction and was lost; three years later the patient complained of a soreness in that region. Upon removal of the calculus it was found to contain a core of cotton. (Courtesy of Dr. John Gunther.)

FIG. 575.—Same case as Fig. 574, after removal of calculus.

ODONTOMAS.

Epithelial Odontomas.—The epithelial odontomas are three in number:

1. Dental root cyst.
2. Dentigerous cyst.
3. Multilocular cyst.

Dental root cysts appear in the roentgenogram as a radiolucent area, sharply defined, and varies considerably in size. (Figs. 467 to 470.)

Figs. 576 to 580.—**Dentigerous Cysts.**

Fig. 576.—Dentigerous cyst in the region of the mandibular canine of a child, aged twelve years.

Fig. 577.—Dentigerous cyst involving the left mandible extending from the premolar region to the middle third of the ramus. Note the molar within the cystic cavity.

Fig. 578.—Dentigerous cyst on the left side of the maxilla involving an impacted left canine.

Fig. 579.—Roentgenogram showing the two impacted canines, the deciduous canines in place, the right and left second incisors being driven out of line by the pressure of the cysts.

Fig. 580.—Dentigerous cyst on the right side of the maxilla involving the right canine.

Figs. 578 to 580.—A bilateral dentigerous cyst in the maxilla of a boy, aged fifteen years.

Note.—Operations by Drs. Ivy and Curtis showed the cysts to extend to the tuberosity of the maxilla, and the floor of each maxillary sinus had been forced upward until the sinuses became obliterated.

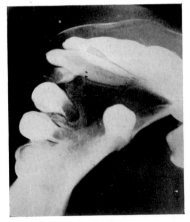

Fig. 576

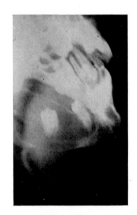

Fig. 577

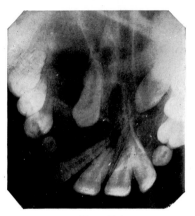

Fig. 578

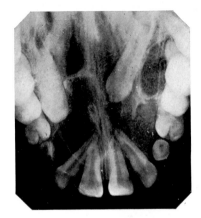

Fig. 579

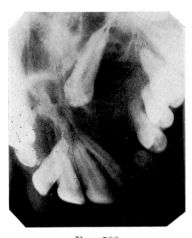

Fig. 580

Figs. 581 to 584.—**Dentigerous Cysts.**

Fig. 581.—Photograph of the dentigerous cyst after its removal. Showing the cyst lining with the coronal portion of the canine extending into the cystic cavity.

Fig. 582.—The outer wall of the cyst after removal. Showing the root of the canine and the attachment of the cyst wall to the tooth.

Fig. 583.—Dentigerous cyst of the mandible of a girl, aged twelve years. The entire ramus is affected, the third molar having been driven backward and upward to the region of the sigmoid notch.

Fig. 584.—Dentigerous cyst of the right mandible causing a pathological fracture.

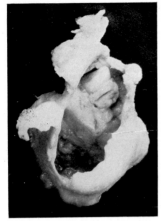

Fig. 581

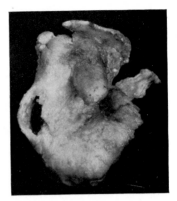

Fig. 582

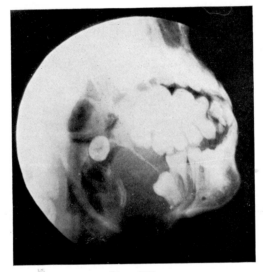

Fig. 583

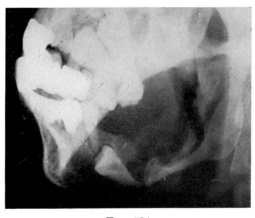

Fig. 584

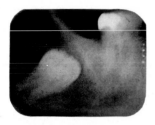 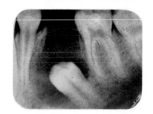

Fig. 585   Fig. 586

Fig. 585.—Dentigerous cyst developing in the region of the mandibular left third molar. The third molar may be seen in the cystic cavity.

Fig. 586.—Dentigerous cyst in the region of the mandibular right second premolar involving the coronal portion of the second premolar.

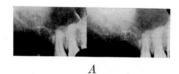

A

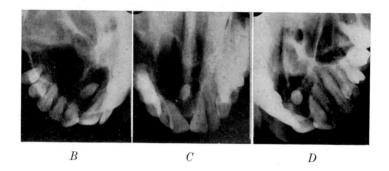

B   *C*   *D*

Fig. 587.—**Dentigerous Cysts.**

Fig. 587.—*A*, two small roentgenograms of the maxillary left molar and premolar regions, showing a radiolucent area over the premolars, but no part of the maxillary sinus. Eastman occlusal film was then used with the result as seen in *B*, *C* and *D*. *B*, left side of the maxilla, showing a supernumerary tooth within a cystic cavity; the cyst extends backward to the tuberosity of the maxilla. *C*, supernumerary tooth shown lying between the first incisors and involved in the cyst. *D*, roentgenogram of the opposite side of the maxilla, showing no pathological condition present in that region.

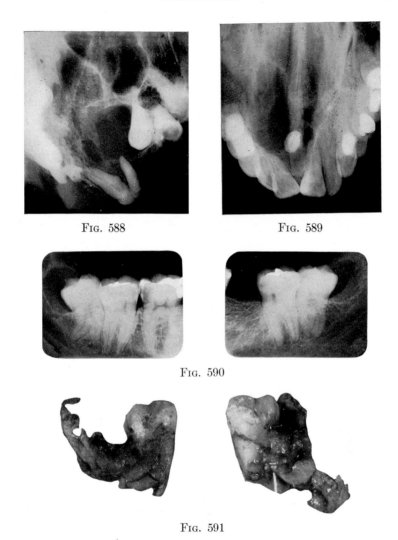

FIG. 588

FIG. 589

FIG. 590

FIG. 591

FIGS. 588 to 591.—**Dentigerous Cysts.**

FIG. 588—Dentigerous cyst involving the maxillary right canine.

FIG. 589.—Dentigerous cyst involving a supernumerary tooth lying in the median line of the palate above the roots of the first incisors.

FIG. 590.—Dentigerous cysts attached to right and left mandibular third molars of patient.

FIG. 591.—Same two teeth (Fig. 590) after extraction, with cystic sacs connected.

Figs. 592 to 596.—**Multilocular Cysts.**

Fig. 592.—Multilocular cyst involving the angle of the mandible.

Fig. 593.—Multilocular cyst involving the premolar and molar region of the maxilla.

Fig. 594.—Multilocular cyst involving the premolar and molar region of the mandible.

Fig. 595.—Multilocular cyst involving the right mandible to such extent as to cause a pathological fracture.

Fig. 596.—Multilocular cyst involving the symphysis of the mandible.

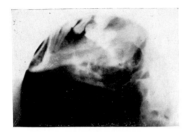

FIG. 592

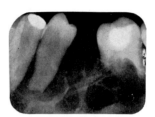

FIG. 593

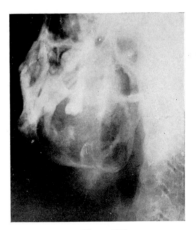

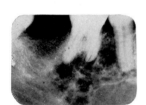

FIG. 594

FIG. 595

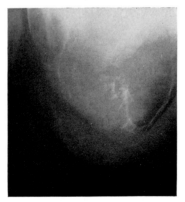

FIG. 596

Figs. 597 to 604.—**Composite Odontomas.**

Fig. 597.—Odontomas between the first and second molar.

Fig. 598.—Same as Fig. 597, localizing the odontoma, showing it to be on the buccal side.

Fig 599.—Large odontoma in the molar region.   This odontoma was on the buccal side.

Fig. 600.—Odontoma in the molar region of the maxilla.

Fig. 601.—Cystic odontoma in the molar region of the mandible.

Fig. 602.—Cystic odontoma in the region of the mandibular canine.

Fig. 603.—Odontoma in the molar region of the maxilla.

Fig. 604.—Odontoma associated with an impacted mandibular canine.

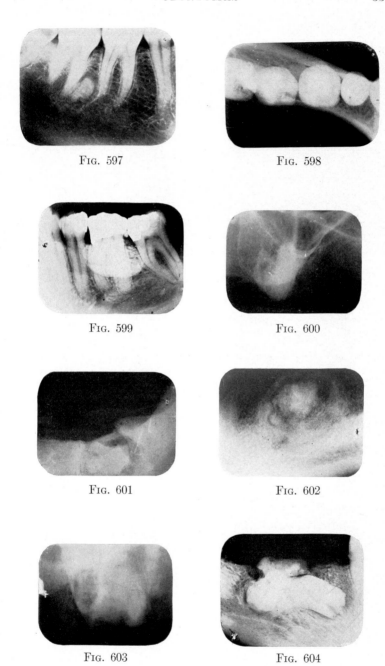

FIG. 597

FIG. 598

FIG. 599

FIG. 600

FIG. 601

FIG. 602

FIG. 603

FIG. 604

22

Figs. 605 to 609.—**Composite Odontomas.**

Fig. 605.—Cystic odontoma located in the molar region of the mandible. Tooth was extracted, the socket failing to heal. Roentgenogram was made revealing the odontome.

Fig. 606.—Odontoma in the region of the maxillary canine.

Figs. 607 and 608.—The right and left side of the maxilla of a woman, aged fifty-four years. There was an exudation of blood on the left side. Roentgenographic examination revealed large odontomas on both sides of the mouth.

Fig. 609.—Roentgenograms of the odontomas after their removal.

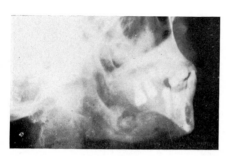

FIG. 605

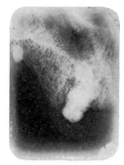

FIG. 606

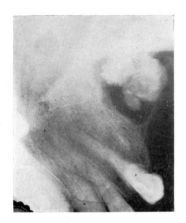

FIG. 607

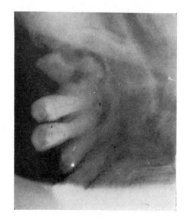

FIG. 608

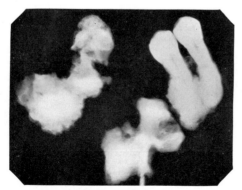

FIG. 609

Figs. 610 to 614.—**Compound Follicular Odontomas.**

Fig. 610.—Compound follicular odontoma in the region of the maxillary left second incisor, the incisor being retained by the odontome and the deciduous tooth.

Fig. 611.—Compound follicular odontoma associated with the impacted canine of the left side of the maxilla.

Fig. 612.—Roentgenogram of the contents of a compound follicular odontoma after removal, showing the tooth-like formations.

Fig. 613.—Cementoma in the apical region of the maxillary left canine.

Fig. 614.—Extra-capsular odontoma, showing a large calcified cauli-flower like mass attached to the coronal portion of the impacte canined.

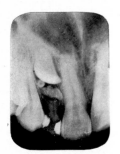
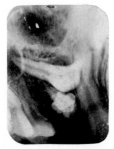
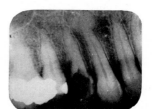

FIG. 610   FIG. 611   FIG. 612

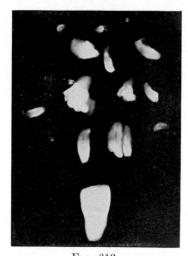

FIG. 613

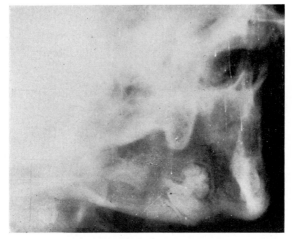

FIG. 614

(341)

The dentigerous cyst is formed by excess fluid secreted between the enamel and the dental capsule, the fluid accumulating and distending the space, and producing a cyst. It is very often called a follicular odontoma and always contains a fully or partially developed tooth or teeth. It appears in the roentgenogram as a large radiolucent area containing one or more teeth. (Figs. 576 to 591.)

The multilocular cyst may arise from abnormal growths of the epithelial "rests" found in diverticula from the enamel organ or from aborted tooth germs. They appear in the roentgenogram as large radiolucent areas with columns of radiopaque bony septa running through the area, and dividing it in a manner to give it the appearance of many cysts. Sometimes the entire growth may undergo osseous changes and appear in the roentgenogram as is seen in Figs. 570 and 592 to 596.

Composite Odontomas.—Composite odontomas originate from aberrations and abnormalities in the development of the whole or part of the constituents of the tooth germ. They appear in the roentgenogram as large radiopaque areas of no definite size or shape. (Figs. 597 to 609.) These odontomas may also be found within a cyst. (Fig. 605.)

Compound Follicular Odontomas.—Compound follicular odontomas originate from an aberration of the dental follicle and appear in the roentgenogram as a large radiopaque area containing numerous denticles. (Figs. 610, 611, 613.)

Extra-capsular Odontocele.—Its origin can probably be explained as being the dental capsule which has undergone a retrogressive metamorphosis. They are very rare. They are seen in the roentgenogram as an impacted tooth with a large radiopaque mass attached to the coronal portion of the tooth. (Fig. 614.)

Cementoma.—Cementoma are either ossification of fibrous odontomas or overgrowth on the part of the osteoblasts in the root membrane. (Fig. 612.)

TORUS PALATINUS.

The first record known of this condition appeared in 1814, when Fox described it as an exostosis of the mid-palatine region. The torus platinus is a hard and solid elevation of the bony palate situated in the median palatine suture and extending to each side of it.

Torus platinus occurs frequently in adults of both sexes, in all ages of life; it varies from a mere uniform crest to a large prominence occupying two-thirds of the palate.

The torus beings to attain an appreciable size after puberty, gradually increasing in size until about the age of thirty years, at

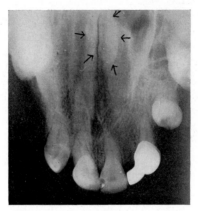

Fig. 615.—Torus palatinus; a radiopaqe area in the median line of the palate in the posterior third.

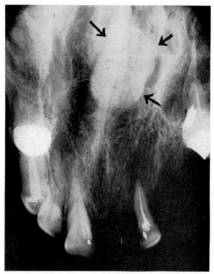

Fig. 616.—The large radiopaque area in the palate is a torus palatinus.

which time growth seems to cease. There may, however, be a change in shape after this period.

It appears on the roentgenogram as a radiopaque area lying in the mid-line of the palate. (Figs. 615 and 616.)

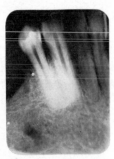

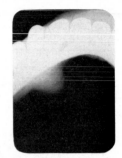

Fig. 617   Fig. 618

Fig. 617.—The radiopaque area between the roots of the first premolar and the canine is the torus mandibularis.

Fig. 618.—An occlusal view of the same case showing the torus on the lingual side of the mandible.

TORUS MANDIBULARIS.

In the region of the canine and premolar teeth at the anterior border of the mylohyoid ridge, it is common to find on the inner plate of the mandible a bulbous extension of varying degrees. It is known as torus mandibularis, and indicated on the roentgenogram as in Figs. 617 and 618.

Figs. 619 to 626.—**Cancellated Structure of the Mandible.**

Figs. 619 and 620.—Illustrating how Nature contributes to the alveolar process to support isolated teeth. Note the radiopaque areas, lines that indicate the reconstruction radiating from the first molar on either side of the mouth.

Fig. 621.—Same as Figs. 619 and 620, except the roots are being absorbed.

Fig. 622.—Same condition existing as in Figs. 619 and 620, except the molar is a non-vital tooth.

Fig. 623.—Sockets formerly occupied by the first molar. The mesial socket is of normal length, while the distal socket is not of normal length due to the absorption of the root having taken place with a subsequent reconstruction of the bone.

Fig. 624.—Large medullary spaces found in the mandible and very often mistaken for some pathological process.

Fig. 625.—Tooth sockets of the first molar, showing the distal socket to be much shorter than the mesial. This is due to the condition as seen in Fig. 626, where one root is absorbed, the bone being reconstructed as in the first molar. Extraction of such teeth without the use of a roentgenogram may easily lead to the belief that the root had been fractured.

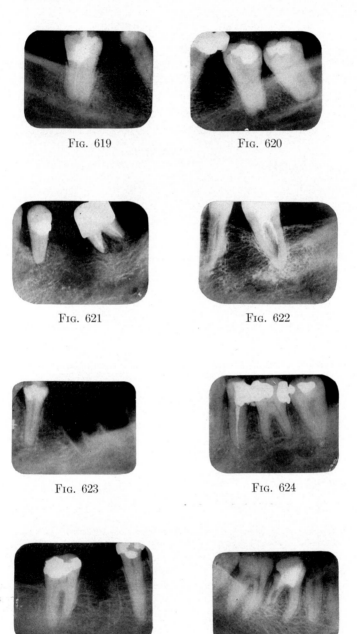

FIG. 619

FIG. 620

FIG. 621

FIG. 622

FIG. 623

FIG. 624

FIG. 625

FIG. 626

CARIES.   (Figs. 627 to 656.)

Caries is undoubtedly the most common of all the diseases of the teeth confronting the dentist, and it is at the same time the most dangerous sign to the patient as well as the most ignored threat to his health.   Unattended conditions may lead to all of the more serious affections attributed to the teeth condition as foci of infection. So it is the duty of the dentist to bend his highest effort to locate any carious condition, to correct it in its incipient stages once it appears.   But, better still, is the prevention of caries by advice as to proper care of the teeth and the elimination of any contributing conditions before it arises.   The prevention of dental decay is the real ideal of the dentist.

No teeth are beyond suspicion of caries no matter what the social, financial, physical condition of the patient, nor how recently under the observation of a dentist who did not make complete clinical and full mouth roentgenologic examinations.   Otherwise there might have been missed recurrent caries under fillings, incipient carious conditions interproximally, caries hidden in the deep fissures of occlusal surfaces.   (Figs. 636, 644 and 648.)

Figs. 627 to 634.—**Caries Indicated by Arrows.**

Fig. 627.—Distally under fillings of the first and second molar.

Fig. 628.—Caries under filling of the mandibular second molar.   Mesially and distally in the first molar, and distally in the second premolar.

Fig. 629.—Caries distally in the mandibular first molar and mesially in the second molar.

Fig. 630.—Caries under filling distally in the mandibular first molar.

Fig. 631.—Caries mesially in the maxillary third molar.

Fig. 632.—Caries buccally in ths mandibular third molar.

Fig. 633.—Caries of the mandibular first molar having involved the pulp as evidenced in the apical region, causing an alveolo-dental periostitis. Caries in the coronal portion of the second molar.   The third molar, which is impacted, shows a carious condition on the occlusal surface.

Fig. 634.—Caries of the second molar on the distal surface caused by the impingement of the impacted third molar.

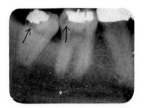

Fig. 627

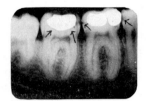

Fig. 628

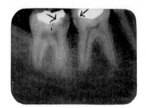

Fig. 629

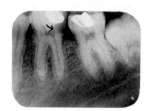

Fig. 630

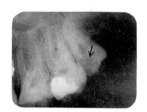

Fig. 631

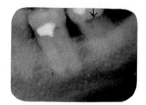

Fig. 632

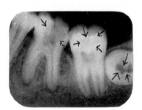

Fig. 633

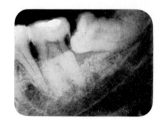

Fig. 634

Figs. 635 to 642.—**Caries.**

Fig. 635.—Caries in the mandibular first molar distally under filling.

Fig. 636.—Caries in the mandibular first, second and third molars. The carious condition is undermining the enamel in the first and third molars. In the second molar the condition exists under a filling.

Fig. 637.—Caries under filling of the maxillary right second premolar.

Fig. 638.—The coronal portion of the tooth is practically separated from the roots by the process of caries. Caries under filling of the mandibular second molar.

Fig. 639.—Caries distally under fillings of the mandibular second premolar and first molar.

Fig. 640.—Abrasion on the labial side of the mandibular canine having the appearance of caries. Caries distally on the first premolar.

Figs. 641 and 642.—Tooth extracted and split in half, showing in Fig. 641 a small filling on the occlusal surface, while in Fig. 642 a large cavity exists.

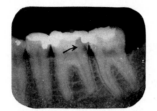

FIG. 635

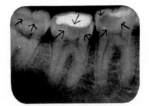

FIG. 636

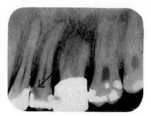

FIG. 637

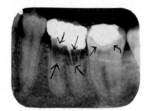

FIG. 638

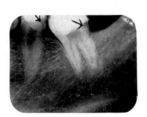

FIG. 639

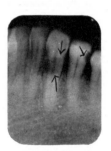

FIG. 640

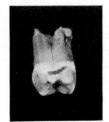

FIG. 641

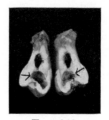

FIG. 642

Figs. 643 to 650.—**Caries.**

Fig. 643.—Caries in the coronal portion of the mandibular second molar.

Fig. 644.—Caries distal half of the mandibular second premolar.

Fig. 645.—Caries on the mesial surface of the inclined mandibular third molar.

Fig. 646.—Caries distally of the maxillary second premolar.

Fig. 647.—Caries mesially in the mandibular first molar. Caries mesially and distally in the retained second premolar.

Fig. 648.—Caries in the crown of the mandibular second molar.

Fig. 649.—Caries in the crown of an impacted maxillary canine.

Fig. 650.—Caries in the crown of an impacted mandibular canine.

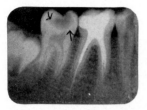

FIG. 643

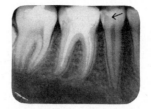

FIG. 644

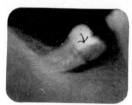

FIG. 645

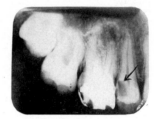

FIG. 646

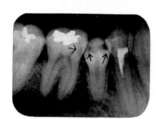

FIG. 647

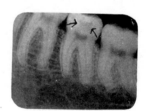

FIG. 648

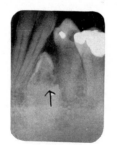

FIG. 649

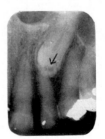

FIG. 650

FIGS. 651 to 656.—**Caries.**

FIGS. 651 and 652.—Two types of film were used in these roentgenograms showing caries: The regular film in which the apical region of the tooth is shown, and the bite-wing film, in which only the coronal portion of the tooth is shown.

FIG. 653.—Caries under filling of the mandibular second molar. Caries under crown of the first molar in which the mesial root is being separated from the tooth.

FIG. 654.—Caries under bridge abutment, with a small piece of tooth structure remaining under the bridge.

FIG. 655.—Distal root of the mandibular molar separated from the tooth by caries.

FIG. 656.—Caries under the shell crown of the maxillary second molar.

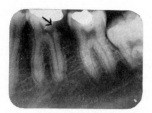

FIG. 651

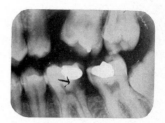

FIG. 652

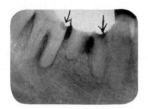

FIG. 653

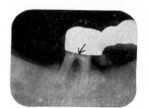

FIG. 654

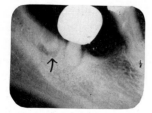

FIG. 655

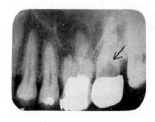

FIG. 656

23

It is recognized that all carious conditions cannot be located merely by clinical examinations, however complete they may be. The roentgenogram plays its most important part in complementing the clinical examination by showing the suspected areas in their relative conditions beyond theory or guess; and an accurate interpretation of the roentgenogram will negate or confirm the conclusions attained clinically. But the interpretation must be accurate.

Definitely to localize caries, if the most perfect result is desired, two distinct types of intra-oral film may be used. One type, the Raper bite-wing film, especially devised for the purpose, has the advantage of allowing both the maxillary and the mandibular teeth to be examined at the same time; but only the coronal portions of the teeth appear in clearness and sufficiency to permit interpretation and localization. Never are the apical regions of the teeth disclosed by this film so as to justify full reliance in diagnosing the presence or absence of caries except in the coronal portions. So we must supplement the use of the Raper bite-wing film by a routine examination of the apical regions of the teeth, and this examination made with the standard intra-oral film, it should be impressed, while not comprehending both the maxillary and mandibular teeth on the same film, will cover on one film the entire coronal and apical portions of the teeth under examination. The Raper bite-wing film is not sufficient in itself for the careful interpreter; the standard film may be; using both to check against each other cannot but give further assurance.

IMPACTIONS.   (Figs. 657 to 688.)

Important as may be the necessity for roentgenographic examinations before any extractions, it should be a mandatory rule in all cases of impactions. This obligation should never be slighted. The possible consequences are too great to risk, and this applies both to operator and patient. Often requiring the utmost skill even with the most positive localization by the roentgenogram, the value of this guide to position, inclination and structure is evident. Those who for years have removed impacted teeth without this assurance can better appreciate not only the greater simplicity in operating but also the release from doubt of the operator and the relief from suffering of the patient.

The illustrations are intended as a brief guide to indicate the various classifications and types of impactions which are met quite regularly, and are meant to serve as suggestions merely of the multifarious examples that may come under observation.

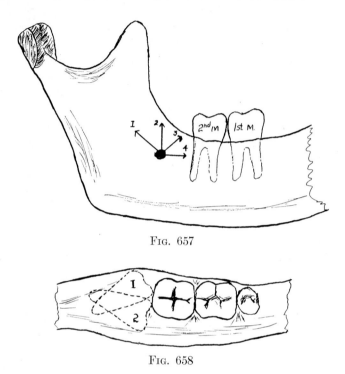

Fig. 657

Fig. 658

Figs. 657 and 658.—Classification of unerupted or impacted third molars. (Thoma.)

Fig. 657.—1, disto-oblique impaction; 2, vertical unerupted; 3, mesio-oblique unerupted; 4, mesio-horizontal impaction.

Fig. 658.—1, lingual displacement; 2, buccal displacement.

They should suggest quite conclusively the unfairness to both the patient and the profession of attempting removals of any impaction without the fullest roentgenographic examinations.

Figs. 659 to 666.—Impaction of the Mandibular Third Molar.

Fig. 659.—Mesio-oblique unerupted mandibular left third molar.

Fig. 660.—Mesio-oblique impaction of the mandibular left third molar.

Fig. 661.—Mesio-horizontal impaction of the mandibular right third molar.

Fig. 662.—Mesio-horizontal impaction of the mandibular left third molar, with pocket surrounding the crown of the tooth.

Fig. 663.—Mesio-horizontal impaction of the mandibular right third molar.

Fig. 664.—Transverse horizontal impaction of the mandibular right third molar.

Fig. 665.—Vertical unerupted mandibular left third molar.

Fig. 666.—Inverted vertical impaction of the mandibular left third molar.

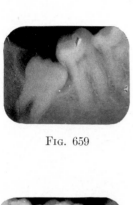

FIG. 659

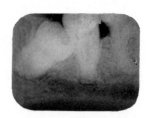

FIG. 660

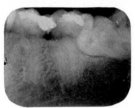

FIG. 661

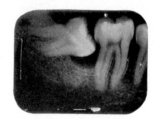

FIG. 662

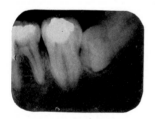

FIG. 663

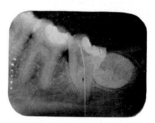

FIG. 664

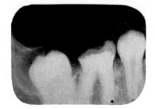

FIG. 665

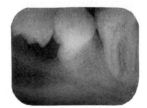

FIG. 666

Figs. 667 to 674.—**Impactions.**

Fig. 667.—An inverted supernumerary tooth inpacted in the region of the mandibular left canine.

Fig. 668.—A supernumerary tooth lying transversely in the maxilla at the apex of the maxillary right first incisor.

Fig. 669.—Lateral view of an impacted mandibular third molar, showing it to be a mesio-horizontal impaction. A roentgenogram is then taken in the vertical plane, the film being placed in the mouth parallel with the plane of occlusion and the rays directed perpendicular to the film through the third molar region, giving the result as seen in Fig. 670.

Fig. 670.—Showing the third molar to be lying in the median line.

Fig. 671.—Lateral view of an impacted premolar.

Fig. 672.—Vertical view of the premolar seen in Fig. 671, showing it to be in the median line of the mandible.

Fig. 673.—Retained mandibular left second premolar inclined lingually.

Fig. 674.—A vertical unerupted mandibular second premolar.

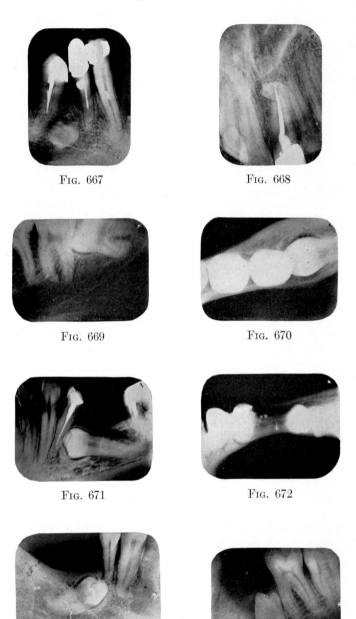

FIG. 667   FIG. 668

FIG. 669   FIG. 670

FIG. 671   FIG. 672

FIG. 673   FIG. 674

Figs. 675 to 682.—**Impactions.**

Fig. 675.—A vertical unerupted, retained mandibular left premolar.

Fig. 676.—An unerupted transversely impacted mandibular right first molar.

Fig. 677.—A retained deciduous molar with a marked absence of the premolar.

Fig. 678.—A retained deciduous second molar preventing the eruption of the premolar.

Fig. 679.—A vertical unerupted maxillary right third molar.

Fig. 680.—A mesio-oblique impaction of the maxillary left third molar.

Fig. 681.—A disto-horizontal impaction of the maxillary right third molar.

Fig. 682.—A disto-oblique impaction of the maxillary right third molar.

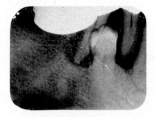

FIG. 675

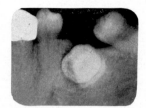

FIG. 676

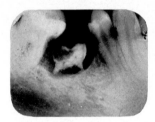

FIG. 677

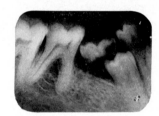

FIG. 678

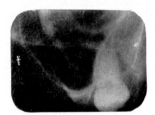

FIG. 679

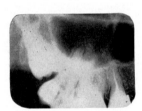

FIG. 680

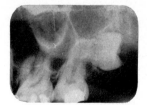

FIG. 681

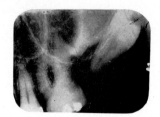

FIG. 682

FIGS. 683 to 688.—**Impactions.**

FIG. 683.—A vertical impacted maxillary right second molar.

FIG. 684.—An impacted supplemental molar, posterior to the maxillary third molar.

FIG. 685.—Vertical unerupted maxillary right premolar.

FIG. 686.—Vertical unerupted maxillary right premolar. These cases clearly demonstrate the great necessity of making a thorough roentgenographic examination prior to any operative procedure where any impaction is involved.

FIGS. 687 and 688.—Vertical unerupted mandibular third molars, with the typical pocket posterior to the crown in which foreign materials, such as food particles, lodge and set up an inflammatory process.

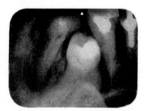

Fig. 683

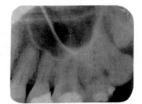

Fig. 684

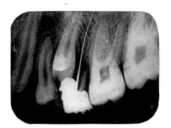

Fig. 685

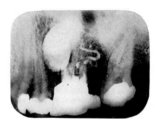

Fig. 686

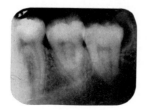

Fig. 687

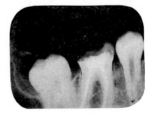

Fig. 688

RESIDUAL ROOTS.   (Figs. 689 to 704.)

The illustrations of residual roots will suffice to warn against a too eager acceptance of even an edentulous mouth as being free of foci of infection, for very often are residual roots found under partial and full dentures that have been worn for years.

Under impression that teeth had been completely removed, these conditions may be too lightly eliminated in seeking sources of troublesome conditions.

Until absolutely sure, the wise practitioner will never attempt any type of restoration; and only after a thorough roentgenographic examination of the oral cavity can we feel sure that any region is entirely free of residual roots.

Figs. 689 to 696.—**Residual Roots.**

Fig. 689.—Residual root of mandibular right third molar lying in the soft tissue.

Fig. 690.—Residual root lying in the maxillary sinus.

Fig. 691.—Residual root of maxillary right first molar lying between the second premolar and second molar.

Fig. 692.—Residual root of mandibular left canine in position associated with a rarefying osteitis with suppuration in the apical region.

Fig. 693.—Apical third of root of the mandibular right second molar within a cystic area.

Fig. 694.—Residual roost of maxillary left first molar in position associated with a cyst.

Fig. 695.—Residual root practically obscured by the shadow of the malar bone.

Fig. 696.—Residual root, as seen in Fig. 695. a different angulation having been used: the malar bone is not superimposed over the root, demonstrating the importance of making more than one roentgenogram when there is any doubt.

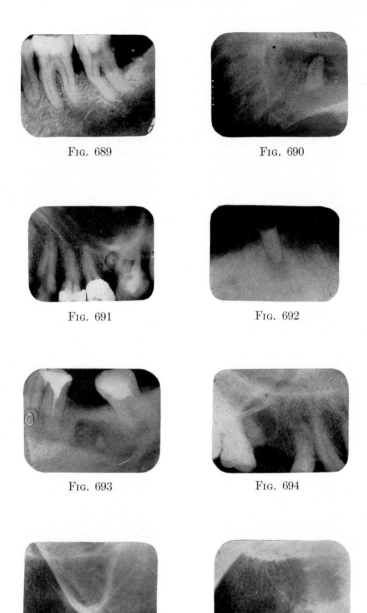

FIG. 689

FIG. 690

FIG. 691

FIG. 692

FIG. 693

FIG. 694

FIG. 695

FIG. 696

Figs. 697 to 704.—**Residual Roots.**

Fig. 697.—Root of the maxillary left first premolar lying in a rarefied area containing granulation tissue.

Fig. 698.—Residual roots of the mandibular left second molar remaining under a bridge.

Fig. 699.—Root fragments in the region of the maxillary left first premolar.

Fig. 700.—Residual root of the maxillary left second incisor.

Fig. 701.—Residual roots of the maxillary right second molar remaining under a bridge.

Fig. 702.—Residual maxillary molar and premolar roots.

Fig. 703.—Residual roots of the maxillary right second molar having the appearance of being in the maxillary sinus. An operation, however, disclosed them to have been lying in the wall of the sinus.

Fig. 704.—Residual root of the mandibular left second premolar remaining under a bridge.

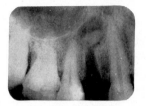

FIG. 697

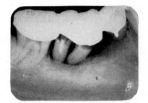

FIG. 698

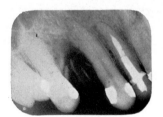

FIG. 699

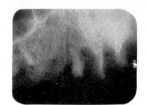

FIG. 700

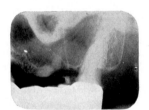

FIG. 701

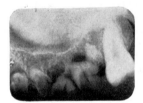

FIG. 702

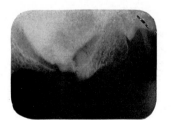

FIG. 703

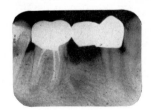

FIG. 704

ROOT-CANAL FILLINGS.   (Figs. 705 to 732.)

No part of dental practice demands a deeper knowledge of anatomy and pathology greater than do cases involving the roots, and especially the apical thirds and surrounding areas. The obviously delicate structural constituency of both the root and the apical foramen, together with the widely different inclinations, sizes, and shapes of roots often discovered in different persons, impresses the importance of this knowledge. Any care less than the utmost that can be employed is lacking in the attention required.

The experienced exodontist is always careful that all bits of tooth structure have been completely removed, taking every precaution by comparing the extracted pieces with his knowledge of the size and structure of the particular tooth even to reconstituting into the whole tooth the broken and splintered particles. So in all removals, fillings, and other operations, the practitioner must account minutely for the material used. The illustrations included here are not exceptional cases; they are only a few of the hundreds that find their way to the active roentgenoglogist, but they answer to point out the lesson intended.

Figs. 705 to 710.—**Root-canal Filling.**

Fig. 705.—Root-canal filling material passing out through the apical foramen of the lingual root of the maxillary right first molar and passing into the maxillary sinus.

Fig. 706.—Gutta-percha point passing out through the apical foramen of the distal root of the mandibular right second molar, continuing through the cancellated bone of the mandible, stopping and turning back when striking the cortical bone at the lower border of the mandible.

Fig. 707.—Root-canal filling passing through the apical foramen of the distal root of the mandibular first molar and communicating with the oral cavity.

Fig. 708.—Root-canal filling passing through the apical foramen into the maxillary sinus.

Fig. 709.—Root-canal filling passing into the maxillary sinus through the apical foramen of the maxillary left first molar.

Fig. 710.—Root-canal of the mandibular right second premolar having its foramen at the distal portion of the apical third of the root and not at the apex of the root.

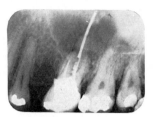

Fig. 705

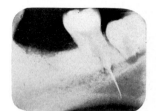

Fig. 706

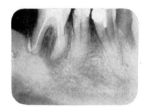

Fig. 707

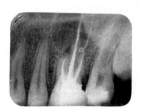

Fig. 708

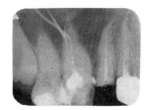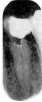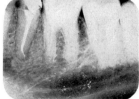

Fig. 709

Fig. 710

24

Figs. 711 to 716.—**Diagnostic Wires, Etc.**

Fig. 711.—Barbed broach used as a diagnostic wire passing a consider-able distance beyond the apex of the tooth, because the patient rarely complains of pain in cases where the diagnostic wire passes beyond the apex.

Fig. 712.—*A*, broken broach in the apical third of the root. *B*, diagnostic wire passing the broken broach.

Fig. 713.—Diagnostic wire passing beyond the apex of the premolar.

Fig. 714.—Broken broach in the apical third of the first premolar.

Fig. 715.—Broken needle remaining after a mandibular injection.

Fig. 716.—Fragment of the metallic backing of the film packet which happened accidentally to be over the emulsion before the exposure was made. In the roentgenogram this shows as a radiopaque line on the film, and was erroneously interpreted as a broken needle.

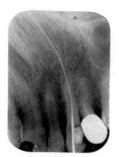

Fig. 711

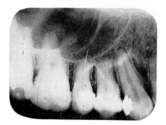
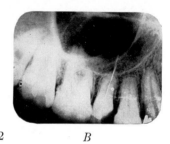

A   Fig. 712   *B*

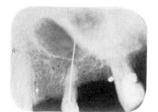
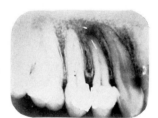

Fig. 713   Fig. 714

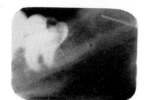
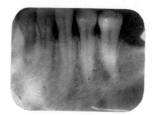

Fig. 715   Fig. 716

Figs. 717 to 724.—**Foreign Objects.**

Fig. 717.—Showing particles of cement filling that were forced down between the periosteum and the bone on the buccal side of the mandible during extraction of the tooth.

Fig. 718.—Same case as Fig. 717 after the cement was removed.

Fig. 719.—Amalgam in the sockets of the premolar teeth. Amalgam filling was placed in the first molar immediately after the removal of the two premolars, the excess of amalgam passing down into the tooth sockets.

Fig. 720.—Fragment of amalgam filling lying in the socket of the mandibular molar.

Fig. 721.—Apical fragment of the maxillary second premolar in position. There was a fistula present. Gutta-percha points were used to locate fragment of root indicated. Upon insertion, points disappeared.

Fig. 722.—Gutta-percha points disclosed, lying in the maxillary sinus. Same case as Fig. 721.

Fig. 723.—Cement in the socket of the mandibular second premolar.

Fig. 724.—Root canal having been filled with soft amalgam, mercury in small quantities has passed through the apical foramen.

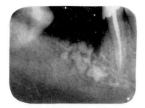

Fig. 717

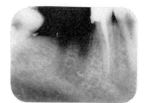

Fig. 718

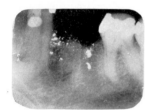

Fig. 719

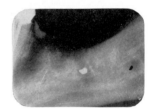

Fig. 720

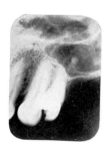

Fig. 721

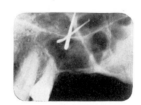

Fig. 722

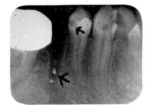

Fig. 723

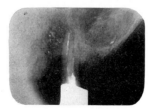

Fig. 724

Figs. 725 to 728.—**Foreign Objects and Fractures.**

Fig. 725 —Amalgam embedded in bone in the region of the first premolar.

Fig. 726.—No root-canal filling was attempted prior to filling the entire tooth with soft amalgam. Excess mercury passed down through the root canal and out into the apical region.

Fig. 727.—A result of faulty technique, the outer rim and hinge-joint of patient's eye-glasses being surperimposed over the maxillary sinus.

Fig. 728.—A result of faulty technique, the roentgenogram having been made with a partial denture in position, obliterating any detail of the alveolar structures.

Figs. 729 to 732.—**Fractures.**

Fig. 729.—Fracture at the neck of the mandibular first molar.

Fig. 730.—Fracture of the mandibule, line of fracture passing below the mesial root of the mandibular first molar.

Fig. 731.—Fracture of the mandible posterior to the third molar. A piece of sequestrum may be seen lying in the line of fracture.

Fig. 732.—Fracture of the maxillary left first incisor at the middle third, held in position by wire ligatures.

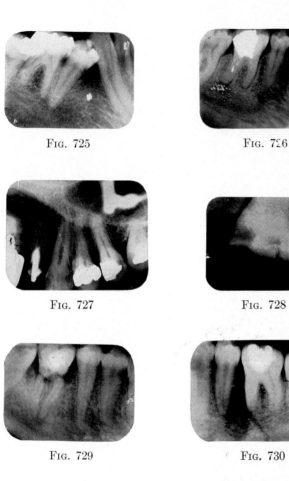

FIG. 725   FIG. 726

FIG. 727   FIG. 728

FIG. 729   FIG. 730

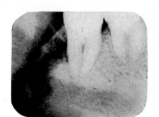

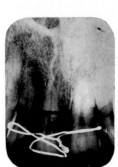

FIG. 731   FIG. 732

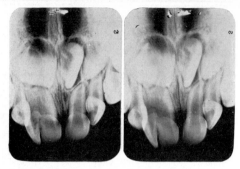

FIG. 733   FIG. 734

FIGS. 733 and 734.—False gemination of the deciduous first and second incisors, the right first incisor being rotated in the maxilla. Patient 2 years of age.

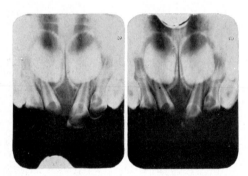

FIG. 735   FIG. 736

FIGS. 735 and 736.—Caries of the maxillary incisors with development of the right second permanent incisor starting, patient one and one-half years of age.

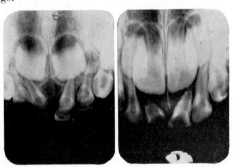

FIG. 737   FIG. 738

FIG. 737.—Caries of the maxillary incisors with development of the right second permanent incisor starting, patient one one-half years of age.

FIG. 738.—The maxillary first deciduous incisors infected, subjecting to unnatural and unfavorable conditions the crowns of the first permanent incisors.

EASTMAN OCCLUSAL FILM. (Figs. 739 to 758.)

The illustrations designate these grosser conditions where the use of the larger film like the occlusal film is necessary. A smaller intra-oral film could not possibly attain the results here secured, could not possibly cover the entire larger lesions with their ramifications, that are so clearly presented.

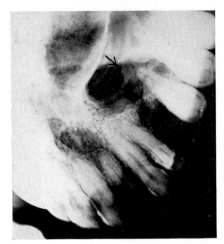 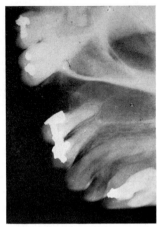

FIG. 739   FIG. 740

FIG. 739.—Root of the maxillary right second premolar lying in the maxillary sinus.

FIG. 740.—Root of the maxillary left first molar lying in the floor of the maxillary sinus over the third molar.

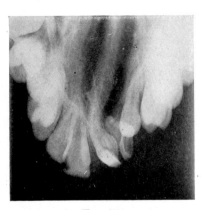 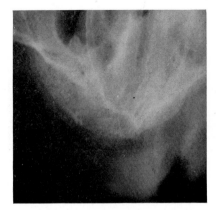

FIG. 741   FIG. 742

FIG. 741.—Cleft palate on the right side of the median line of the palate, showing a dilaceration of the right first incisor.

FIG. 742.—Necrosis of the maxilla in the region of the maxillary left canine.

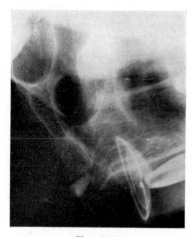

Fig. 743

Fig. 744

Fig. 743.—Eye-glasses superimposed over the maxilla.

Fig. 744.—Condensing osteitis in the region of the maxillary right premolar.

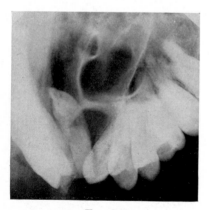
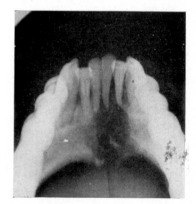

Fig. 745

Fig. 746

Fig. 745.—Cleft palate with a loss of the right second incisor, the right first incisor being inverted.

Fig. 746.—Fracture of the mandible in the region of the symphysis involving the four incisor teeth.

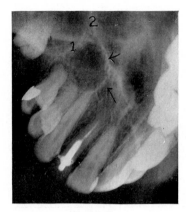
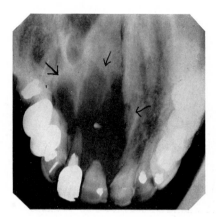

FIG. 747   FIG. 748

FIG. 747.—Infected cyst over the second premolar, separated from the maxillary sinus by the bony septum (1), indicating (2) the dividing line between the maxillary sinus and the nasal fossa.

FIG. 748.—Large cyst involving the anterior portion of the palate.

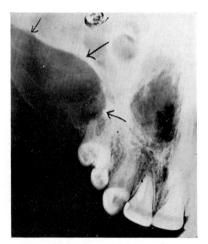

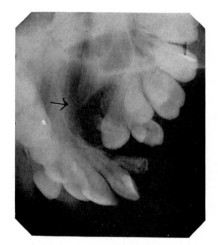

FIG. 749   FIG. 750

FIG. 749.—Large cyst involving the maxillary left molar region.

FIG. 750.—Cleft palate involving the right second incisor, the canine being impacted.

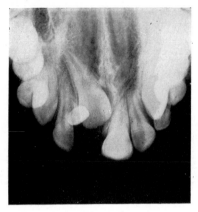 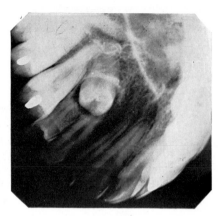

Fig. 751   Fig. 752

Fig. 751.—Supernumerary tooth causing a deflection of the maxillary left first incisor.

Fig. 752.—Impaction of the maxillary left second premolar.

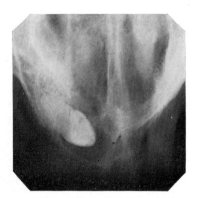 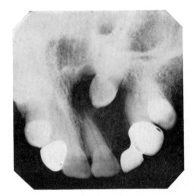

Fig. 753   Fig. 754

Fig. 754.—Dentigerous cyst, involving the canine tooth in an edentulous mouth.

Fig. 753.—Dentigerous cyst involving the maxillary right canine.

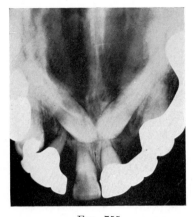 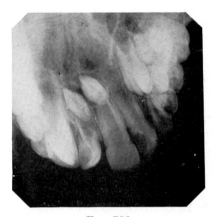

FIG. 755   FIG. 756

FIG. 755.—Bilateral impaction of the canine teeth.

FIG. 756.—Two supernumerary teeth lying in the palate posterior to the maxillary first incisors.

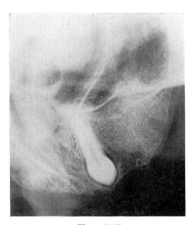 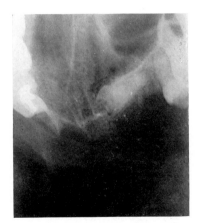

FIG. 757   FIG. 758

FIG. 757.—Impacted maxillary right canine.

FIG. 758.—Impacted maxillary right canine, showing an absorption of the coronal portion of the tooth.

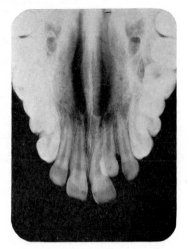

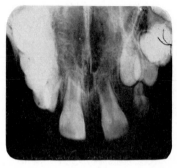

Fig. 759   Fig. 760

Fig. 759.—A curving and deflection of the maxillary right first incisor
prevents the complete eruption of the second incisor.

Fig. 760.—Congenital absence of the right maxillary second incisor.

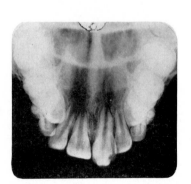

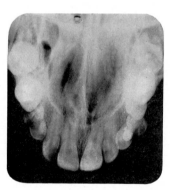

Fig. 761   Fig. 762

Fig. 761.—Supernumerary tooth superimposed over the right first incisor.

Fig. 762.—Congenital absence of the right and left permanent canines.

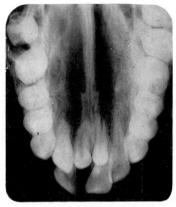
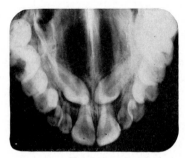

FIG. 763   FIG. 764

FIG. 763.—Two supernumerary teeth causing a deflection of the first incisors.

FIG. 764.—Congenital absence of the maxillary second incisors and impactions of both maxillary canines.

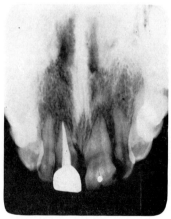

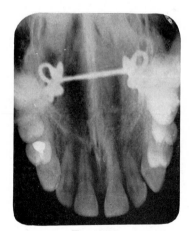

FIG. 765   FIG. 766

FIG. 765.—False gemination of the maxillary right first and second incisors.

FIG. 766.—Bridge of eye-glasses superimposed over the palate.

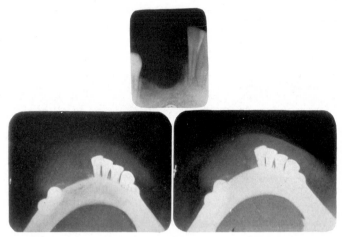

Figs. 767 and 768.—Epulus or fibroma in mandibular left canine and incisor region. By shorter exposure we obtain the outline of the tumorous mass and bone, if present, as in this case, becomes evident.

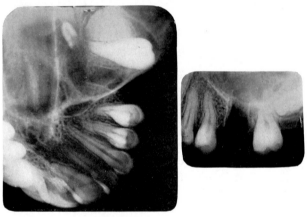

Fig. 769   Fig. 770

Figs. 769 and 770.—Demonstrating the necessity of the occlusal film. Fig. 769 reveals a root in the sinus, while the small intra-oral film of the same case, Fig. 770, fails to show the root.

LEONTIASIS OSSEA.   OSTEOMYELITIS.   (Figs. 771, 772, 773.)

Rather remarkable roentgenograms, showing very clearly condi-tions that rarely confront the average practitioner, but such cases should at least be recognized by the experienced roentgenoglogist when they do appear, so that proper reference to the oral surgeon or physician may be made with some definite understanding of the conditions.

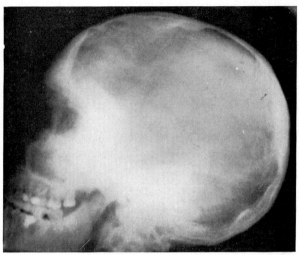

Fig. 771.—Leontiasis ossea. Lateral view of the head, showing a radi-opaque area in the sphenoid bone.

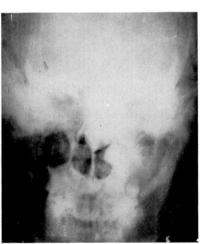

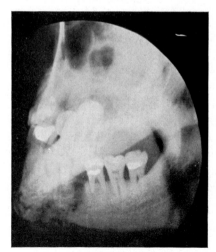

Fig. 772   Fig. 773

Fig. 772.—Leontiasis ossea. Anterior-posterior view, showing the radi-opacity to be on the right side of the head.

Fig. 773.—Osteomyelitis of the mandible in the region of the symphysis.

25

CHAPTER X.

LOCALIZATION OF ROOT CANALS AND FISTULOUS TRACTS BY USE OF LIPIODOL.

THE function of the roentgenologist in the diagnosis of root-canal conditions cannot be over-emphasized. Not only does the roentgenographic examination confirm the clinical determination as to the existing lesions and other pathological appearances, but after surgical or general treatment the roentgenogram is the only dependable check-up.

Root-canal treatment requires an extremely intimate perception of the most minute affections, extreme caution in procedure, a delicate tenchique in operations, an abundance of patience.

Dependence upon the diagnostic wire in root-canal therapy has always presented objectionable features. No matter how careful the operator, there always impends the threat of the wire passing through the apical foramen and penetrating the tissue structures of the apical region. Introduction of infection thereby is no rare result. Nor is it strange that infection does occur often. The true and actual shape and size of the root canal under treatment may not be completely realized by the use of the wire. This must be conceded; for the great number of troublesome conditions arising consequent to treatment are indisputable proof. Wires hopelessly embedded in a cavity beyond the possibility of removal except by delicate surgery are not unusual. Many cases of extraction and root amputations are attributable to this factor. But however remote the possibility of complications may seem, the dentist does not close his eye before any distant danger nor risk any future threat that may be avoided. That is why we remove the diagnostic wire so promptly after completing the tests; for, sealed with the soft and malleable material employed in the operation, undue pressure and pounding upon it must be prevented.

Search to secure a safer method and to eliminate the danger due to the diagnostic wire has been going on rather continually. Experiments have progressed sufficiently to indicate the possible discarding of the use of the wire in most cases of root-canal explorations. The

(386)

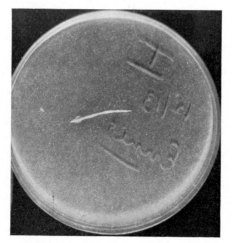

FIG. 774.—Incubated agar plate, photographed twelve hours after application, shows cotton-point saturated with lipiodol. Discloses absence of germicidal quality in lipiodol. Experiments prove a germicidal neutrality in lipiodol, the fluid neither inhibiting nor exciting the growth of bacteria. Adding camphorated monochlorphenol in varying portions confirms not only the property of radiopacity inherent in lipiodol, though decreased by dilution, but it also indicates the quality of sterilization.

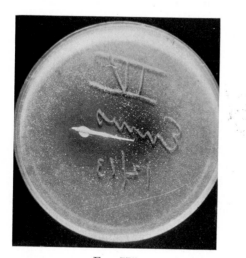

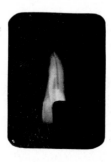

FIG. 775   FIG. 776

FIG. 775.—Photographed after use of a solution composed as follows: lipiodol, 1 part; camphorated monochlorphenol, 2 parts.

FIG. 776.—Note the greatly lessened radiopacity, reduced because of the dilution of the lipiodol to a point approaching inefficiency.

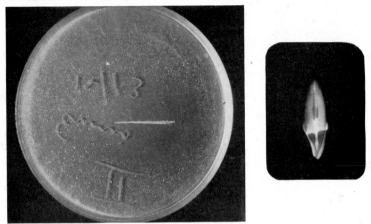

Fig. 777   Fig. 778

Figs. 777 and 778.—Indicates an increase in radiopacity, the sterilizing quality of the solution remaining practically unchanged. The proportions of the solutions used here are: lipiodol, 4 parts; camphorated monochlorphenol, 1 part.

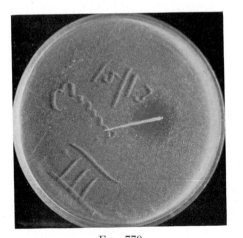 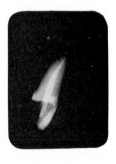

Fig. 779   Fig. 780

Figs. 779 and 780.—Where the solution used is formed of: lipiodol, 16 parts; camphorated monochlorphenol, 1 part. The radiopacity is further increased and the sterilizing qualities fully adequate for root-canal exploration.

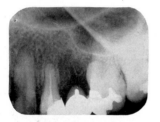 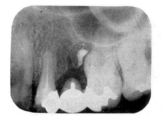

Fig. 781   Fig. 782

Figs. 781 and 782.—Localization of Fistulous Tract.

Fig. 781.—Roentgenogram of case prior to injection of lipiodol. Clinically, there was a fistula with suppurative discharge; but roentgenogram did not definitely reveal location of pathological lesion.

Fig. 782.—Same case after injection of lipiodol, shows fistulous tract leading to mesial buccal root of first molar.

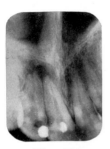 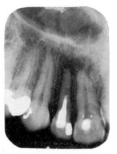

Fig. 783   Fig. 784

Fig. 783.—Maxillary second left incisor failed to respond to treatment.

Fig. 784.—Lipiodol worked into root canal by means of paper point. Note stoppage at middle third of root.

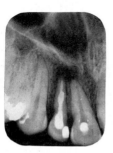 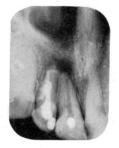

Fig. 785   Fig. 786

Figs. 785 and 786.—Lipiodol injected by Luer syringe passed further into canal, roentgenograms taken at different angles reveal a mesial perforation of the root.

newer method suggests a simpler technique, a saving of time, and a surer system of securing truer knowledge of conditions.

Instead of the diagnostic metallic wire being employed as the agent whereby the roentgen-ray is used to determine the length and configuration of the root canal, and to ascertain whether access

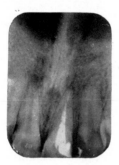 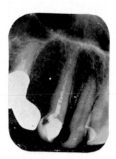

FIG. 787   FIG. 788

FIGS. 787 and 788.—Roentgenograms showing root canals filled with lipiodol.

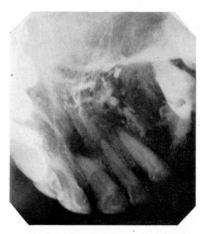

FIG. 789.—Roentgenogram showing large cyst with lipiodol in the cyst cavity. Clinically there was a discharging sinus in the premolar region.

to the apical foramen has been attained, superior results may be achieved by the proper use of the paper point, the paper point being saturated with lipiodol diluted with camphorated monochlorphenol.

Lipiodol, a non-irritant, sterilized, radiopaque fluid, may be injected into the roots without causing any pain to the patient. It has been extensively and successfully used for general roentgeno-logic work in the medical field, especially in connection with lesions of the gall-bladder.

"Lipiodol, an iodized vegetable oil, is the product of the intimate combination of red-poppy oil with pure metalloid iodine, without any trace of chlorine." These words are quoted *verbatim* from the descriptive circular issued by the manufacturer.

As the radiopacity of the lipiodol becomes reduced by dilution, care must be exercised to add just the proper proportion of cam-phorated monochlorphenol; for, naturally, radiopacity lessens in proportion to the amount of the dilution.

TECHNIQUE OF INTRODUCTION.

To introduce lipiodol into lesions of the mouth for diagnostic purposes requires a careful and definite technique; for particular care must be exercised to insinuate the fluid into the area under examination and to prevent any excess of the fluid remaining in the oral cavity outside the lesion. Otherwise, this excess may appear on the roentgenogram so as to mislead the interpreter.

Root-canal Technique. — Two methods offer for introducing lipiodol into root canals. By one method, a paper point (Johnson and Johnson) may be dipped into the fluid, and then, with the small excess of fluid that will easily adhere to the point, the point is carried into the root canal with a slow-pumping movement. Care-fully executed, the lipiodol will be carried into the apical region of the tooth and will adhere to the walls of the canal; and the point may be sealed in the canal with gutta-percha. Any excess lipiodol should be removed from the external surface of the crown.

Lipiodol may also be injected into root canals by means of a Luer syringe. After grinding a steel needle to a blunt point, a small amount of lipiodol is placed in the syringe and the blunted needle attached. Enough unvulcanized rubber to fill the cavity of the tooth is placed around the needle, the needle then carried to the opening of the root canal and the unvulcanized rubber surrounding the needle pressed tightly in the cavity. A slight pressure on the syringe releases the lipiodol into the root canal. Withdrawing both needle and attaching rubber, a paper point saturated with the lipiodol solution is inserted into the canal and sealed. A roent-genogram will reveal the outline of the canal clearly. (Figs. 780, 785 and 787.)

Cystic Technique.—Lipiolol solution injected into the fistulous tracts of the mouth goes to the seat of the lesion and aids in revealing on the roentgenogram the exact outlines of the tract. It may be injected into the tracts by the use of the Luer syringe and blunt needle as employed when treating root canals, a large piece of unvulcanized rubber being placed surrounding the needle, the needle inserted into the tract, and the rubber passed down over the needle to close the orifice of the tract. Slowly injecting the lipiodol into the tract until the lesion is full, this being indicated by the back-flow of the excess fluid, the needle is removed and the opening closed with an unvulcanized rubber plug.

The roentgenogram may then be made, the tract appearing as a radiopaque area leading to the seat of the lesion. (Figs. 781 and 782.)

Care of Syringe and Needle.—The syringe and needle should never be used without having been first thoroughly sterilized by boiling. Especially with the needle must this never be neglected. It must be boiled; never flamed; for the combustion of the oil constituent in lipiodol leaves minute particles of carbon in the lumen of the needle, and at the same time the iodine, thus liberated, attacks the metal.

INDEX.

A

ABSCESS, chronic, 268–272
  periosteal, 299
Absorption, alveolar process, 296
    horizontal, 303
    vertical, 302
  of teeth, 312
    external, 313
    internal, 321
    odontolysis, 312
    osteolysis, 312
Acute exacerbation, 288, 289
Adventitious dentine, 306
Agenesia, 270
Alopecia, 56, 57
Alveolar process, absorption of, 296
    horizontal, 303
    vertical, 302
Alveolo-dental periostitis, 277
Ampère, 43
Anatomical landmarks, 207
  alveolar structures, 209
  anterior palatine foramen, 215
  coronoid process, 219
  external oblique ridge, 267
  genial tubercles, 254
  hamular process, 217
  in relation to roentgenology, 207
  malar bone, 219
  mandibular canal, 253
  maxilla, 209, 210
  maxillary sinus, 221
  median suture, 217
  medullary spaces, 254
  mental, foramen, 255
    ridge, 254
  mylohyoid ridge, 267
  nasal cartilage, 209
    fossa, 210
  nasolacrimal canal, 252
  nasopalatine canal, 210, 211
  nutrient canals, 255, 260
  premaxillary suture, 217
  teeth, 209–267
  temporomalar suture, 221
  tuberosity of maxilla, 217
Angulation chart, 86
  frontal sinuses, 117
  horizontal, 81, 82, 96
  mandibular, canine, 94
    incisors, 95
    molars, 91, 92
    premolars, 93

Angulation chart, maxillary, canines, 89
    incisors, 90
    molars, 84, 85
    premolars, 87, 88
    sinuses, 116, 117, 120
  rules governing, 75
  vertical, 86, 88, 89, 90
Anode construction, 36
Anterior palatine foramen, 215
  posterior distortion, 61, 62
Apparatus, 66, 72
  Ritter dental, 70, 71, 72
  Victor C. D. X. mobile type, 67, 68, 69
Auto-transformer, 45

B

BITE–WING, film, 108, 109
Bone, cancellated structure of, 253, 344
  regeneration, 302, 314, 345
Broken instruments, localization of, 167

C

CALCAREOUS degeneration of pulp, 308
    complete calcification, 308
    nodules, 308
    partial calcification, 308
Calcification of pulp, complete, 308
  partial, 308
  of teeth, 132, 134
Calculus, 323, 327
Cancellated structures of bone, 344
Canine, mandibular, angulation of, 94
  maxillary, angulation of, 89
Caries, dental, 136, 346, 352
    children, 376
Cassettes, 174
  holders for, 151, 152
Cathode, construction of, 38
  stream, 32
Cementoma, 342
Cementum, hyperplasia of, 322
Cieszynski's rule of isometry, 76, 77
Clark's technique, 163, 164
Classification of impactions, 355
Cleft palate, 378, 379
Composite odontomes, 338
Compound follicular odontomes, 342
Condensing osteitis, 302
Construction of films, 176

Coolidge tubes, 39, 66
    anode construction, 36
    cathode construction, 38
    exhausting, 38
    tungsten filament, 33
    types, 39
Coronoid process of madible, 219
Current, 43
    alternating, 43
    direct, 43
Cysts, dental root, 327
    dentigerous, 327
    multilocular, 327, 334

D

DARK-ROOM equipment, 185, 186, 187, 188
    practical hints for, 193, 195
Deciduous teeth, 132
Degeneration of pulp, 308
Density of anatomical structures, 272
Dental pathology, 272
    acute localized infection, 272
    chronic infection, 272
    cysts, 291
    exacerbation, 272, 286
    lesions, types of, 274
    periapical lesions, 274
    peridental absorption, horizontal, 299
        gingivitis, 299
        lesions, 296
        vertical, 302
    periostitis alveolo-dental, 274
    rarefying osteitis, 277, 279
    stages of, 291
    suppuration, 287, 288
    root cysts, 327
Dentigerous cyst, 327
Dentine, adventitious, 306
    senile, 307
Dermatosis, roentgen-ray, 54, 193
    cause of, 54
    chronic, 55
    effects of, 55, 56, 57
    idiosyncrasy for, 59
    stages of, 54, 55
    treatment of, 58
Developer, care of, 187, 189
Developing, 177
    reducing, 177, 192
    solutions, 177
        factoral method, 189
        fixation chemistry of, 176, 180
        reduction chemistry of, 182
        temperature of, 184
Development, chemistry of, 177, 178
Developmental crypt, 135
Diagnostic wires, 370
Dilaceration, 308

Diphyodontic gemination, 310
Distortion, 73, 74
    anterior-posterior, 77, 78
    longitudinal, 77, 78
Dosage, erythema, 59
    treatment, 58

E

EASTMAN occlusal film, 130
Electrical terminology, 43
Electron, characteristics of, 42
    presence determined by, 41
    production of, 42
    supply, 40
Enamel tubercles, 276
Epithelial cell rests, 290
    odontomas, 327
    sheath of Hertwig, 290
Epulus, 384
Equipment, apparatus, 70, 71, 72
    dark-room, 185, 186, 187, 188
Erythema dose, 59
    treatment, 58
Exacerbation, 288, 289
Examination of oral cavity, 196
        periodic, 143
        time for, 138
Exposures, 82
External absorption, 313
    oblique ridge, 261
Extra-capsular odontome, 342
Extra-oral films, 109
        of frontal sinus, 117
        of lateral head, 113, 114
        of malar process, 124
        of mandible, 109, 110, 112
        of maxillary sinus, 117, 118
        of sphenoidal sinus, 121, 122
        of temporomandibular articulation, 111, 112, 115, 116
    technique of, 73, 109

F

FALSE gemination, 310
Faradic current, 196, 197
    pulp tester, 196
Fibroma, 384
Filament, cathode, 47
    transformer, 44
Fillings, root-canal, 368, 370
Film holders, 129
    holding of, 60
Films, bite-wing, 108, 172
    chemistry of, 176
    construction of, 131, 176
    developing of, 177
    extra-oral, 109, 172
    fixation, 180

Films, insertion of, for mandibular canines, 128
    incisors, 129
    molars, 127
    premolars, 127
  maxillary canines, 126
    incisors, 126
    molars, 125
    premolars, 125
  intra-oral, 171
  mounting of, 172
  occlusal, 177
  placement of, 126, 129
  reduction, 177
  washing of, 183
Fixation, chemistry of, 180
Fluoroscopy, 60
Follicular odontomes, 340, 342
Foramen, 212
Foreign objects, 372
Fractures, 378
  of jaw, 73
  of teeth, 375
  zygomatic process, 122, 124
Frontal sinuses, 116, 117, 120

G

Gagging, cause of, 130
  prevention of, 131
Gemination, 310, 376
  diphydontic, 310
  false, 310
  true, 310
Genial tubercles, 254
Gingivo-alveolo-dental periostitis, 299

H

Hamular process of sphenoid bone, 217, 218
Head, position of, 75, 76, 77
Holders, film, 129
Horizontal absorption, 303
  angulation, 81, 82, 83
  plane, 74, 75
Hyperplasia of cementum, 322

I

Idiosyncrasy, 59
Illumination, 205
Immobilization, 160
Impacted teeth, localization of, 166
Impactions, 354
  classification of, 355
Incisors, mandibular, angulation of, 95
  maxillary, angulation of, 85, 90
Intensifying screens, 173

Internal absorption, 321
Interpretation, 202
  requisites, 73
Intra-oral films, 171

J

Jaws, fractures of, 73

K

Kearsley stabilizer, 46, 52
Keratosis, 55
Kilowatt hour, 43

L

Landmarks, anatomical, in relation to roentgenology, 207
Le Masters' technique, 86, 87, 100
Leontiasis ossea, 384
Lipiodol, 386
  care of syringe, 392
  cystic technique, 392
  root-canal technique, 391
  technique of introduction, 386
Localization of broken instruments, 167
  of maxillary canine, 163
  of root fragments, 167
  of teeth, 96, 158
  of third molar, 166
Longitudinal distortion, 77

M

Malar bone, 219
  landmarks of, 221
Mandible, anatomical landmarks of, 253
  occlusal plane of, 78
  structure of, 344
Mandibular canal, landmarks of, 263
  canine, angulation of, 94
    insertion of film, 128
  incisors, angulation of, 95
    insertion of film, 127
  molars, angulation of, 91
    insertion of film, 92, 127
  premolars, angulation of, 93
    insertion of film, 127
  third molars, localization of, 166
Maxilla, landmarks of, 209
  occlusal plane of, 77, 78
  tuberosity of, 217
Maxillary canine, angulation of, 89
    insertion of films, 126
    localization of, 163
  incisors, angulation of, 90
    insertion of film, 126

Maxillary canine, molars, angulation of, 84, 85
    insertion of film, 87, 125
  premolars, angulation of, 87
    insertion of film, 88, 125
  sinus, 221
    abnormalities of, 229
    alveolar extension of, 225
    anatomical variations of, 226, 235, 236
    blood supply of, 250, 251
    differential interpretation of, 241
    infra-orbital extension, 227
    nutrient canals of, 247, 251
    palatine extension of, 227
    recession of, 239
    relation of teeth to, 239
    septa of, 224, 240
    tuberosity, extension of, 227, 233
Median suture, 212, 217
Medullary spaces, 253
Mental foramen, 255
  landmarks of, 257
  ridge, landmarks of, 254
    variations of, 253
Metol dermatitis, 193
Miller's technique, 165, 166
Milliampère, 43
Molars, mandibular, angulation of, 91, 93
  maxillary, angulation of, 85, 86
Mounting, 172
Mounts, 173
Multilocular cysts, 327, 335
Mylohyoid ridge, 267

N

Non–calcification of roots, 267
Nutrient canals, mandible, 255
  maxilla, 250

O

Occlusal film, 130, 172, 377
  plane, 75, 78, 79
    leveler, 80
    of mandible, 105
      floor of mouth, 107
      symphysis, 106
    of maxilla, 100
Odontolysis, 313
Odontomas, composite, 337, 338
  compound follicular, 340, 342
  epithelial, 327
  extra-capsular, 341
Ohm, 43
Ohm's law, 43
Oral cavity, examination of, 196
Orientation, line of, 78, 96, 99

Os zygomaticum (see malar bone), 219
Osteitis, chronic, rarefying, 277
  etiology of, 277
  roentgenographic abnormalities, 277
  symptoms of, 277
  with cyst formation, 291
  etiology of, 291
  roentgenographic abnormalities, 291
  symptoms of, 291
  with granulation tissue, 279
  etiology of, 279
  roentgenographic abnormalities, 279, 291
  symptoms of, 279
  with suppuration, 288
  etiology of, 288
  roentgenographic abnormalities, 288
  symptoms of, 288
  condensing, 302
Osteolysis, 312
Osteomyelitis, 384
Osteo-alveolo-dental periostitis, 299
Osteoradionecrosis, 64

P

Palate, landmarks of, 211, 215
Pathology in relation to roentgenology, 272
Penetration, 96
Periapical bone lesions, 169, 170
  dental lesions, 274
    localization of, 169, 170
Peridental absorption, horizontal, 303
    vertical, 302
  gingivitis, 299
  lesions, 296
Periosteal abscess, 299
  etiology of, 299
  roentgenographic findings of, 300
  symptoms of, 300
Periostitis, alveolo-dental, 296
Photographic materials, chemistry of, 176
Placement of film in children, 157
Planes, occlusal, 75, 78, 79
  sagittal, 75, 78, 79
Power, 43
Premaxillary suture, 212
Premolars, mandibular, angulation of, 93
  maxillary, angulation of, 85, 87
Pulp, calcification of, 306
  complete, 308
  partial, 308
  degeneration of, 308
  nodules, 308
  tester, 196

R

RADIATION test, 59
Radiolucent area, 207, 273
Radiopaque area, 207, 273
Rarefying osteitis, chronic, 277, 279
    with cyst formation, 291
    with granulation tissue, 279
    with suppuration, 288
Reducing, 177, 182
Reduction, chemistry of, 182
Regeneration of bone, 302
Residual roots, 364
    localization of, 167, 168
Resistance, 43
Roentgenograms, identification of, 175
Roentgenographic examinations, 273
    results of, 22
Roentgenography, intra-oral, 77
    extra-oral, 73
Roentgenologic qualifications, 67
Roentgenology for children, 132
    extra-oral, 140
    intra-oral, 141, 142
Roentgen-ray burn, 54
    dermatosis, 54
    diagnostic value of, 272
    discovery of, 15, 16
    erythema dose, 59
    idiosyncrasy, 59
    penetration, 43
      point, mandible, 98
        maxilla, 96
    production of, 40, 42
    protection from, 59
    quality, 42
    radiation, 42
      tests for, 41, 59
    transformer, 44
    tubes, 32, 33
    voltage requirements of, 44
Root-canal filling, 368
    localization of, 386
Roots, non-calcification of, 276
    residual, 369
Rotary converter, 47

S

SAGITTAL plane, 74, 75, 77, 78
Salivary calculi, 323, 326
Screens, intensifying, 173
Senile dentine, 307
Septa of maxillary sinus, 224, 225, 240
Sheath of Hertwig, 291
Sialoliths, Wharton's duct, 323
Sinuses, frontal, 116, 117, 120
    maxillary, 221
Sphenoid, hamular process of, 217
Sphenoidal, 121, 122

Static, registration of, 175
Step-down transformer, 45
Step-up transformer, 49
Stereoroentgenography, 158
    angulation, 161
    examination, 161
    immobilization, 160
    method of exposure, 162
    placement of film, 158
Supernumerary teeth, 137, 146, 380

T

TANKS, developing, 187
Technique, Clark's, 163, 164
    bite-wing, 108, 109
    children, 153, 155
    extra-oral, 109
    frontal sinuses, 116
    lateral head, 109, 110, 112
    mandible, 109
    maxillary sinuses, 117, 118
    regions examined, 109
    sphenoidal sinus, 123, 124, 125
    temporomandibular articulation, 109, 111, 115, 116
    zygomatic process, 125
    intra-oral, horizontal, 74, 75, 77
      vertical plane, 76
    Le Masters, 86, 87, 100
    Miller's, 165, 166
    occlusal film, 100
      children, 148
      mandible, 105
        floor of mouth, 107
        symphysis, 105, 106
      maxilla, 100
        canine, 102
        maxillary sinus, 103, 104, 105
        molar, 103
        palate, anterior, 100
Teeth, calcification of, 132, 134
    deciduous, 132
    developmental crypt, 135
    fractures of, 375
    impacted, localization of, 166
    investing tissue of, lesion of, 296
    localization of, 163, 166
    retained, 144, 145
    vitality test, 196
Temperature, developing, 184
Temporomalar suture, 220
Temporomandibular articulation, 109, 111, 115, 116
Terminology, electric, 43
Thermal test, 201
Tonsilliths, 323
Tooth development, 267
Torus, palatinus, 342
    mandibularis, 344

Transformers, 44
  filament, 47
  primary circuit, 44
  secondary circuit, 44
  step-down, 45
  step-up, 44
Transillumination, 201
True gemination, 310
Tube movement, horizontal plane, 74, 75, 80, 81
  vertical plane, 74, 75, 83
Tubercles, enamel, 276
  genial, 254
Tuberosity of maxilla, 218, 219

Tumors, 73

V

VICTOR roentgen-ray, 69
Vitality test, 196
  technique for, 198
  thermal, 201
Volt, 43

W

WASHING, chemistry of, 183
Watt, 43
Wharton's duct, 107